Teaching Technologies in Nursing and the Health Professions

Wanda E. Bonnel, PhD, GNP-BC, ANEF, is associate professor at the University of Kansas School of Nursing, where she has taught for over 20 years. Currently, she teaches graduate-level courses in teaching with technologies, foundations in education, and teaching strategies, creating a learning environment, among others. She is a fellow in the National League for Nursing (NLN) Academy, the recipient of the Kemper Teaching Award at the University of Kansas, and the Sigma Theta Tau Regional Pinnacle Award for Computer-Based Professional Education Technology. Dr. Bonnel has been the primary investigator on five funded grants and research projects, including Best Practices in Feedback to Online Students and Online Course Feedback, What Do We Mean? (both funded by NLN). She has published more than 25 peer-reviewed articles and contributed 6 invited chapters to edited works, the majority of which have focused on aspects of nursing education. A certified geriatric nurse practitioner, Dr. Bonnel is a grant reviewer for NLN and Health Resources and Services Administration, an editorial board member of the *Journal of Gerontological Nursing,* and a manuscript reviewer for the *International Journal of Nursing Education Scholarship* and the *Journal of the American Academy of Nurse Practitioners.*

Katharine Vogel Smith, PhD, RN, is associate professor and assistant dean for program evaluation at the University of Missouri, Kansas City, where she has taught since 1991. Dr. Smith's research has included 17 funded grants, most of which focused on some aspect of teaching, advanced education, and nursing traineeships. Professional presentations include international and national posters and oral presentations focusing on simulation and ethical issues related to health care. Dr. Smith is published primarily in the area of nursing ethics and serves as a consultant editor for *Nursing Ethics: An International Journal for Health Care Professionals.* Her clinical nursing career has focused on cardiovascular nursing, including clinical nurse specialist work in cardiac rehabilitation.

Teaching Technologies in Nursing and the Health Professions

Beyond Simulation and Online Courses

WANDA E. BONNEL, PhD, GNP-BC, ANEF

KATHARINE VOGEL SMITH, PhD, RN

SPRINGER PUBLISHING COMPANY
New York

Springer Publishing Company, LLC
11 West 42nd Street
New York, NY 10036
www.springerpub.com

Acquisitions Editor: Margaret Zuccarini
Senior Editor: Rose Mary Piscitelli
Cover design: David Levy
Composition: Laura Stewart, Apex CoVantage, LLC
Ebook ISBN: 978-0-8261-1848-6

10 11 12 / 5 4 3 2 1

The author and the publisher of this Work have made every effort to use sources believed to be reliable to provide information that is accurate and compatible with the standards generally accepted at the time of publication. Because medical science is continually advancing, our knowledge base continues to expand. Therefore, as new information becomes available, changes in procedures become necessary. We recommend that the reader always consult current research and specific institutional policies before performing any clinical procedure. The author and publisher shall not be liable for any special, consequential, or exemplary damages resulting, in whole or in part, from the readers' use of, or reliance on, the information contained in this book. The publisher has no responsibility for the persistence or accuracy of URLs for external or third-party Internet Web sites referred to in this publication and does not guarantee that any content on such Web sites is, or will remain, accurate or appropriate.

Library of Congress Cataloging-in-Publication Data

Teaching technologies in nursing and the health professions : beyond simulation and online courses / [edited by] Wanda E. Bonnel, Katharine Vogel Smith.
    p. ; cm.
  Includes bibliographical references and index.
  ISBN 978-0-8261-1847-9 (alk. paper)
1. Nursing—Study and teaching. 2. Medical education. 3. Educational technology. I. Bonnel, Wanda E. II. Smith, Katharine Vogel.
  [DNLM: 1. Education, Nursing—methods. 2. Computer-Assisted Instruction—methods. 3. Education, Nursing, Continuing—trends.
4. Educational Technology—trends. 5. Internet. WY 18 T2533 2010]
  RT71.T346 2010
  610.73076—dc22   2010000411

Printed in the United States of America by Bang Printing

Contents

SECTION I: CONCEPTS FOR TEACHING AND LEARNING ACROSS DIVERSE TECHNOLOGIES

SECTION II: FACULTY AS LEARNING FACILITATORS WITH TECHNOLOGY

Contributors
Evidence-Based Review Abstracts

Chapter 2 Keeping Up With Changing Technology, Self-Directed Learning, and Lifelong Learning

Evidence-Based Review Abstract:
Online Readiness to Learn
Jamie S. Myers, RN, MN, AOCN
Doctoral Candidate, University of Kansas School of Nursing, Kansas City, KS

Chapter 3 Theory and Teaching Technologies

Evidence-Based Review Abstract:
Learning to Learn With Concept Mapping
Patricia Conejo, RN, MSN, WHNP
Assistant Professor of Nursing, Avila University School of Nursing, Kansas City, MO

Chapter 4 Technology Teaching and Lesson Planning

Evidence-Based Review Abstract:
Best Practice for Orienting Students to Learning
Suzanne Stricklin, MSN, RN
Assistant Professor, Miami University Nursing, School of Engineering and Applied Science, Oxford, OH

Chapter 8   Technologies and Active Learning

Evidence-Based Review Abstract:
Storytelling as a Teaching and Learning Concept
Cheryl A. Spittler, MSN, RN, CEN, CPSN
Patient Care Coordinator, Quinn Plastic Surgery Center, Overland Park, KS

Chapter 9   Feedback, Debriefing, and Evaluation With Technology

Evidence-Based Review Abstract:
Reflective Journaling
Janet Reagor, RN, MS
Assistant Professor of Nursing, Avila University School of Nursing, Kansas City, MO

Chapter 10   Online Education and Diverse Teaching and Learning Opportunities

Evidence-Based Review Abstract:
Seeking Best Evidence, Promoting Online Integrity
Amanda L. Alonzo, PhD, RN
Lecturer, Pittsburg State University, Pittsburg, KS

Chapter 11   The Changing Classroom and Technology

Evidence-Based Review Abstract:
Listening for a "Click" in Classrooms
Shelley D. Barenklau, CRNA, MS
Clinical Assistant Professor, University of Kansas School of Allied Health,
Nurse Anesthesia, Kansas City, KS

Chapter 12   Simulation and Clinical Learning

Evidence-Based Review Abstract:
Faculty Orientation to Learning Simulation
Christine L. Hober, MSN, RN, C
Assistant Professor, Fort Hays State University, Hays, KS

Contributors
Case Examples

Chapter 14   Pedagogy, Technology, and Clinical Education

Exhibit 14.1   Case Example:
Online DNP Preceptor Studio
Diane Ebbert, PhD, ARNP, FNP-BC
Assistant Professor, Director, Advanced Practice Programs, University of Kansas
School of Nursing, Kansas City, KS

Moya Peterson, RN, MS, CPNP, ARNP, PhD
Assistant Professor, University of Kansas School of Nursing, Kansas City, KS

Exhibit 14.2   Case Example:
Pocit Videos: Point-of-Care Instant Teacher
Mary N. Meyer, RN, MSN, ARNP
Clinical Assistant Professor, University of Kansas School of Nursing, Kansas City, KS

Sharon Kumm, RN, MN, CCRN
Clinical Associate Professor, University of Kansas School of Nursing, Kansas City, KS

Reviewers

Heidi Boehm, RN, MS
Unit Educator, Family Medicine, Orthopedics, The University of Kansas Hospital, Kansas City, KS

Marie Collins, RNC, BSN
Clinical Informatics, St. John's Mercy Medical Center, St. Louis, MO

Lindsey Montello, MSN
Consultant, Shawnee, KS

Nancy Mosbaek, PhD, RN
Education Specialist, Kansas State Board of Nursing, Topeka, KS

Kathleen Neff, MA
Research Associate, University of Missouri–Kansas City, School of Nursing, Kansas City, MO

Peggy Ward-Smith, PhD, RN
Associate Professor, University of Missouri–Kansas City, Kansas City, MO

Judith Wilkinson-Hiam, PhD, RN
Author/Consultant, Shawnee, KS

Foreword

Teaching technologies are ubiquitous, and using technology for teaching in nursing is inescapable. In most nursing classrooms, students are actively engaged in learning using computers and classroom response systems. In many learning resource centers, students learn clinical decision making by enacting scenarios with human patient simulators. In the clinical setting, students find information for care plans from textbooks on their handheld electronic book readers, and might review a vodcast of a procedure prior to performing it. And, beyond the classroom, students use social networking, collaborative tools, Twitter, and text messaging to be continuously in touch with their faculty, classmates, and other resources to support their learning. It is in this context that *Teaching Technologies in Nursing and the Health Professions: Beyond Simulation and Online Courses* arrives as a timely resource to provide guidance to nurse educators about how to use these technologies in their own courses and educational programs.

This book, unlike others that explain technical aspects, focuses instead on how to integrate the technologies into teaching and to use them to facilitate student learning. Organized around best practices such as promoting active learning, respecting students' diverse ways of learning, fostering collaboration among the students, and providing rich and rapid feedback, this book provides clear directions for using a variety of teaching technologies.

In this book, nurse educators will find resources for attaining curriculum goals of integrating health information technology, informatics, and information literacy into the curriculum; harmonizing generational differences among students with varying abilities to use technology; developing self-directed learners; and assuring that all students learn how to acquire and use information necessary for clinical practice. Of particular interest is the emphasis on the use of health information technologies for enhancing patient care, clinical decision making, and promoting patient safety.

Novice and experienced nurse educators will find practical information grounded in theory and evidence. The links to resources, guided reflection, learning activities, and questions for further thought in each chapter prompt the reader to consider how best to use the technologies, while evidence-based reviews offer clear examples of how to integrate the technologies discussed in chapters into a lesson plan.

Nurse educators have a responsibility to prepare the next generation of nurses to use technologies to assure quality patient care and to be lifelong learners. *Teaching Technologies in Nursing and the Health Professions: Beyond Simulation and Online Courses* will help nurse educators do just that.

Diane M. Billings, EdD, RN, FAAN
Chancellor's Professor Emeritus
Indiana University School of Nursing
Indianapolis, IN

Preface

Whether working with students at a distance, in the learning lab, or class-rooms and clinical settings, educators can use varied technologies to enhance student learning. Technology helps us prepare our students, update our staff, and keep our patients safe. Nursing is a clinical profession, and technology is a part of our work, as well as that of future generations. Health information technology has been described as a top priority for improving health care, with goals specific to informing clinical care, interconnecting clinicians, personalizing care, and improving population health. With this rapidly increasing technological environment, we are at a point where all educators need to be comfortable with technology.

New generations of students are part of a technology-savvy world and are familiar and comfortable with technology. Faculty have the opportunity to maximize these student strengths, using technology to help students create meaning in complex clinical education. Major organizations, including the National League for Nursing and American Association of Colleges of Nursing (AACN), have called for faculty to prepare students in technologies. Strategies for teaching both with technology and about technology are incorporated in this text.

Whatever the teaching setting, a key concept is making a good fit between the student learning objectives, assignments, and selected technology tools. This text provides frameworks to help in decision making, providing enough direction to guide decisions and plans, but appreciating that further learning resources will be needed to keep up with rapidly changing technology. Strategies for advancing our skills to stay a step ahead (or keep up with) our learners are included.

OVERVIEW OF TEXT ORGANIZATION

This book is conceptualized in three sections. The first section provides an overview of teaching and learning concepts that have relevance across a variety of technologies and introduces the Integrated Learning Triangle for Teaching With Technologies. Chapter 1 reminds readers of the basics of good teaching practices and blends those practices with technology. Since the cutting-edge technology of today will quickly be replaced by newer technology, concepts of self-directed learning and lifelong learning are reviewed in Chapter 2. In Chapter 3 readers are introduced to concepts and theories that guide teaching with technology and capture significant student learning. Lesson plans are considered in Chapter 4 as tools for integrating technology to build on students' current knowledge, make content relevant, help students apply content, and evaluate learning. With the rapid proliferation of readily available text-based, audio, and video resources, Chapter 5 considers student computer skills and information literacy, now a critical competency in all nursing programs.

Section II assists readers in enhancing their faculty skills as learning facilitators with technology. Basic communication functions with technologies, especially text-based communication, are addressed in Chapter 6. Clinical implications, including the important role that technology plays in safe patient care, are incorporated. Chapter 7, acknowledging that learning communities consist of groups of people engaged in common learning goals, provides facilitator strategies and faculty tools to help diverse students learn with technologies. Chapter 8 considers the authentic learning that can be a part of learning with technology, providing opportunities to bring the world to students via online opportunities and applied assignments. The faculty role in providing student feedback, as well as debriefing intense learning experiences, is described in Chapter 9. Evidence suggests that feedback and debriefing are critical in technology-rich environments, helping deepen and cement student learning.

Section III guides faculty in considering that principles of good teaching serve across technologies. Chapter 10 addresses online education with its many unique teaching and learning opportunities. The changing classroom and technology are discussed in Chapter 11. Technology provides a means by which to increase faculty teaching opportunities with all classroom students, whether in traditional or distant settings. Chapter 12, addressing simulated clinical learning experiences, focuses on teaching methods required to help students apply critical thinking and safety competencies, skills needed to provide safe care in today's fast-paced health care settings. Chapter 13 focuses on helping students become excited about using clinical technologies such as electronic health records (EHRs) to promote patient safety and care quality. Chapter 14 is about teaching clinical technologies, focusing on faculty tools to guide students in safe, efficient use of clinical technologies and accompanying caring behaviors.

The final chapter, Chapter 15, discusses ongoing faculty learning needs and pedagogical issues for the future. Opportunities for using technology projects to further scholarship and continue work with interdisciplinary teams are emphasized.

Throughout the text, applications specific to online, classroom, and clinical teaching technologies are shared. These topics have relevance for both student development, staff development, and even patient education and the Internet. The Institute of Medicine (IOM) Health Professions Competencies are integrated in chapter discussions, as well as technology recommendations from AACN, National League for Nursing, and other national groups.

FORMAT AND FEATURES

This text is designed for graduate students, faculty, and staff educators learning to use technologies effectively and efficiently in their teaching. Based on educational theory and best practices, the text integrates resources from a variety of disciplines. The text begins with broad teaching and learning concepts that have relevance across a variety of technologies. Guided by a chapter goal, each chapter is organized in a time-efficient format with brief text, bullets, and resource exhibits. Readers learn not just one technology but tools for using a variety of new technologies. Since faculty come from varied teaching settings, with unique resources and diverse student levels, concepts in this text are presented broadly for faculty to adapt to their own teaching and learning milieus. The following features are included.

Reflective Questions

Each chapter begins and ends with reflective questions to support our faculty roles as reflective educators seeking to improve our teaching. Introductory reflections are designed to acknowledge and build on readers' past experiences. Ending reflections are designed for self-reflection on new ideas gained from reading and plans for using these ideas.

The Integrated Learning Triangle for Teaching With Technologies

A major feature of the text is the Integrated Learning Triangle for Teaching With Technologies. Designed to provide a central organizing tool for lesson planning and decision making, the Integrated Learning Triangle serves as a faculty guide for determining if and how technology can promote student learning. Accompanying questions help address planning needs. Whether technology decisions are for an entire course or one assignment, the Integrated Learning Triangle applies across a wide variety of educational and practice technologies from low to high technology.

Chapter Resources and Case Examples

Each chapter provides a variety of resources. Selected chapters include self-assessment tools, case examples, and further resources to promote learning to teach with and about technologies.

Quick Tips

Each chapter ends with quick teaching tips to serve as reminders of important concepts for planning and implementing our teaching and learning activities.

Evidence-Based Review Abstracts

Since our focus is teaching and learning with the best evidence, many chapters provide an evidence summary of a pedagogical concept with references synthesized to highlight best educational practices. For example, topics such as student readiness to learn and promoting online integrity are included.

Online Resources for Further Learning

Since this text supports lifelong learning, each chapter includes Web sites for gaining additional teaching and learning ideas. While Web addresses for important resources are supplied throughout each chapter, URLs may change, so readers are reminded to perform a search by site name or reference to identify a changed address.

Questions for Further Reflection

These questions serve as prompts for ongoing discussions with colleagues. The questions also provide opportunities to consider unique issues or topics for a specific setting.

In this text, the broad term *technology* encompasses diverse technologies in clinical and classroom settings, in addition to Web-based learning tools. Additionally, the authors use the words *faculty* and *we* interchangeably since both authors continue along with our readers in the teaching with technologies journey.

Nurses have unique roles in using technology both in learning and in caring for patients. The rapid increase in online learning, the call for all undergraduate students to gain informatics competencies, and the rapid increase in high-fidelity patient simulator use are all examples of need for faculty to update their skills in technology. This book is designed to help readers appreciate the rapidly changing future of technology and clinical practice, refocusing on the need to be self-directed, lifelong learners. As the authors' own children, truly technology-savvy learners, advance in their educational careers, the authors are often reminded of the important roles faculty play in helping students to be successful. We hope our readers gain ideas for using technology in promoting success of many future students!

Wanda E. Bonnel
Katharine Vogel Smith

Acknowledgments

We wish to thank our families for their patience as we pursued this writing project; individuals who have contributed resources and shared reviews for various chapters; our university colleagues for introducing us to many technology resources; and our Springer colleagues, especially Margaret Zuccarini, for her encouragement in text development.

Concepts for Teaching and Learning Across Diverse Technologies

SECTION
I

1   What Does It Mean to Teach With Technology?

CHAPTER GOAL

Gain an overview of teaching with technologies, including an introduction to the text and tools that will be used throughout the book to promote teaching and learning with technology.

BEGINNING REFLECTION

1. What experiences have you had teaching with technology?
2. What are your current goals for expanding the use of technology in promoting student learning?

INTRODUCTION

Traditional teaching methods have not always kept up with the rapidly changing world of technology. Rapid expansion in online learning, national calls for all students to gain informatics competencies, and the major impact of high-fidelity patient simulators all support the need for faculty competence and confidence in teaching with technologies.

As all levels of faculty seek to enhance traditional teaching with technologies, how do nursing faculty keep up with the rapid changes? This book provides an overview of teaching and learning concepts, or pedagogies, that are relevant across a variety of technologies. This book can help new or seasoned educators gain strategies for keeping up with technologies. It can also help them make thoughtful selections of how and where technology should be integrated into learning environments to meet specific educational goals. Readers can gain new ideas for integrating technology-based learning strategies in their own teaching projects.

Technology and the changing clinical arena are an interesting mix. Addressing technology is important in this time of rapid change in health care and renewed emphasis on safety and quality in clinical care. As national reports document problems with communication and safety in the health professions, technology can provide unique opportunities for making improvements in these critical areas. What considerations are necessary in technology integration into health care programs? How does technology affect teaching and learning? Basic approaches that will be covered in this text include the following:

- Helping our students (and ourselves) recognize personal learning styles and skills for self-directed learning.
- Gaining a conceptual toolkit that can promote success in teaching/learning concepts (such as evidence-based practice) with a technology base.
- Gaining familiarity with a variety of available teaching resources such as the Quality and Safety Education for Nurses (2009) project.
- Gaining a template for teaching technologies based on best practice evidence.

This book is about combining the best of the traditional teaching and learning principles with new, rapidly changing technologies. Theories such as that of adult learning can help us do this. We will explore the advantages and limits of teaching with and about technologies. We do not expect our readers to become experts in all technologies. Rather, the idea of the book is to understand good, basic teaching principles and apply them to rapidly changing technologies. This book is not intended to develop skill proficiency with a particular software or technology, but rather to introduce pedagogical concepts and practices relevant to future teaching with technology.

Methods supplied throughout this text are consistent with adult learning theory. In rapidly changing arenas such as educational technology and clinical knowledge, there are benefits to time-tested theory in guiding rapid decision making to meet student and patient needs. This is particularly important for students in clinical professions.

WHY ARE PEDAGOGIES IMPORTANT AND WHAT DO THEY MEAN?

A world of technology has opened up for our use in teaching and learning. In particular, our overall focus on pedagogies has been enhanced by the major shift that online learning has presented. As learning moved online, educators were pushed to think about what they were trying to accomplish with teaching rather than just moving a classroom session to the Web. As new technologies have emerged for both classroom and clinical units, more opportunities to consider pedagogy and technology combinations exist. While the term *andragogy* was defined as referring specifically to adult learners (Knowles, 1984), the more common umbrella term of *pedagogy* will be used throughout this text. A pedagogical approach reminds us to keep student learning at the forefront. While there are varied definitions for *pedagogy*, the term relates to the activities of educating or instructing that facilitate learning by another. The concept of facilitator will be key throughout our discussions.

Additionally, best practice pedagogies relate to learning by doing. While definitions of best practice can vary, examples of teaching principles and resources based on evidence include the following:

- Chickering and Gamson (1987). This classic reference describes seven best practices for teaching.
- Carnegie Mellon University (2009). In this recent report, research-based principles are expanded to include both teaching and learning principles.
- Commission on Behavioral and Social Sciences and Education (1999). This resource provides a basic reference on how people learn.

Technology enhances teaching opportunities and in some cases may even make teaching easier. Technology, for example, allows ready access to new materials. Gaining knowledge of Alzheimer's Association resources at one time required making phone calls or trips across town to the association office to gain print copies of learning materials. Now these materials are readily accessible online. The question then becomes how to help students know where to look to gain these best tools not only now but also into their future practice. If we help students identify appropriate resources such as the Alzheimer's Association, they will be able to act as self-directed learners, using these resources in the future.

Current approaches to teaching with technologies are quite varied. The meaning of even a seemingly straightforward term such as *online course* can vary greatly. Our intent is to build opportunities and enhance readers' repertoire of tools for conveying content and using technology when it presents the best solution for helping our students learn. As faculty, we want not only to convey content to our students but also to help them understand what to do with the content, so they can make the connections between concepts and put concepts into context. Determining the best practices to do this is a worthy goal.

WHAT DO WE MEAN BY *TECHNOLOGIES?*

Technology is a very broad term, and its use in education has been described in different ways. Skiba, Connors, and Jeffries (2009) have considered the term to consist of three frames including educational technology, information management, and clinical practice technology. While there is overlap in the three frames, they provide direction for our discussions. We will be addressing our teaching from the educational technology frame, and considering how best to teach concepts within the practice frame with an overarching information literacy theme.

While we are privileged to live in a technology-rich time with all the accompanying opportunities, this fast and furious pace may lead us to question how we can make teaching with technologies manageable. Since technology changes too fast to constantly focus and learn all technology updates, we are reminded to focus on the broad concepts or pedagogies that facilitate our use of technologies to promote student learning.

Educational Technologies

Technology provides educational options. We are talking not only about teaching online but also about the many ways that classroom and clinical activities can be enhanced by technology. For example, we can give students the option of reading texts in print versions or using online electronic text or chapters to guide a class such as the online *Retooling for an Aging America* (Institute of Medicine [IOM], 2008). Also, assignments traditionally shared in the classroom, such as creating posters or brochures for

Exhibit 1.1

HOW MANY WAYS ARE THERE TO TEACH RESPIRATORY ASSESSMENT?

- Should all classes on respiratory assessment be taught the same way? As you think about your experiences or further teaching plans, is technology needed to teach respiratory assessment?
- Could technology enhance learning on this topic?
- How can the Integrated Learning Triangle for Teaching With Technologies, introduced in this chapter, guide you in making decisions about what approaches work best for your students and setting?

health fairs, can be developed electronically and viewed electronically. Students can view these documents prior to the class and come ready to debrief in class or at an online discussion. Using this electronic medium not only works for students but also helps prepare them for using these resources as tools in their clinical practice. We will be thinking about our resources, courses, and assignments differently. We will be using theories and best practices to guide us when research does not keep up with our rapidly changing needs.

Even in our core or basic classes, there are many opportunities for using technology to enhance teaching and learning. In a classroom pathophysiology class, for example, faculty might use technologies to capture self-assessments, present automated quizzes with instant feedback for student learning, apply case studies to make the learning more relevant, engage students with questions embedded in PowerPoint presentations, and assign a relevant clinical project such as teaching handouts or posters to be completed with technology. Follow-up discussions at online discussion boards might be assigned. The nice thing is that good teaching principles have a good match with technology. See Exhibit 1.1, "How Many Ways Are There to Teach Respiratory Assessment?"

Information Management and Clinical Practice Technology

We are taking on new roles as we move into teaching technologies in the clinical setting. Technology has populated our clinical worlds in terms of managing information and working with our patients. Four broad technology goals for practice, conveyed in the health information technology report by Health and Human Services (2004), are specific to informing clinical care, interconnecting clinicians, personalizing care, and improving population health. Practice technology not only includes teaching students to care for patients on respirators in the intensive care unit but also involves changes from paper to electronic patient charting or documentation. Health care professionals gain unique information about populations via electronic data sets. Additionally, technology provides opportunities to promote clinical safety, support population health, gain efficiency in teaching and learning, and makes it easier for health professionals to track information, get reminders on care issues, and develop plans for positive patient outcomes.

The IOM safety reports remind us to use technology for a variety of reasons, including enhanced team communication to promote patient safety and outcomes. Patient safety, in common practices such as medication administration and fall prevention, is now often promoted with technologies that help assess, monitor, and direct care planning. Faculty gain opportunities to help students use technology in new ways to support patient care. Gaining familiarity with diverse technologies for teaching and learning in order to promote safe student practices and positive patient outcomes will be a focus in this text.

The overarching information literacy theme has particular relevance to our students of the future, serving as a basic platform for all of their professional work. Information literacy serves as a guide to faculty for teaching evidence-based practice. As faculty we first consider where to find best evidence to share with our students and then teach them how to find their own best evidence for their future practice.

OUR DIVERSE LEARNERS AND THEIR CLINICAL PRACTICE

We will be working with diverse students in the classroom and in the clinical units, including students who are diverse both in their cultural backgrounds and in their learning styles and interests. Our students bring a range of academic proficiencies as well as unique talents and desires to become clinical professionals. As faculty we are challenged to help all of our students gain learning tools for success. An outcomes orientation in nursing education also includes a focus on the student remediation that technology makes much easier for us to provide.

We are preparing to teach students who will be practicing across diverse settings from acute care to homes to long-term care. Students provide care ranging from health promotion to palliative care. The amount of information they will need can seem overwhelming, unless we use broad concepts to help students learn the must-know content.

THINKING CONCEPTUALLY

Our discussions in this text will often relate to the broad concepts that can help us organize information and move forward with diverse patient populations, rapidly changing times, and technologies. We are preparing to teach students who will be practicing across diverse settings from acute care to extended care settings and caring for patients from infants to frail elders. Thinking conceptually helps us keep track of broad content areas. Concepts remind us quickly of what we already know about a topic area and lay a foundation for further learning and organizing.

Concepts and themes addressed in this text will include teaching about being professional and ethical, using evidence, thinking critically, and being competent in clinical skills. The rapidly changing field of genetics and genomes is one example. Students need to understand the basic concepts of genetics and technology for patient testing and treatment purposes. Beyond their basic clinical skills, counseling and supporting will be called into play. Much of their work in this area will relate to having good ethical models for decision making and for patient support strategies, along with an awareness of psychosocial issues and professional practice models.

BUILDING OUR TOOLKIT WITH MODELS AND RESOURCES TO GUIDE

Technology, if used in the best ways, presents opportunities to facilitate many aspects of teaching and learning. Theories and best evidence can guide our pedagogies. Adult education reminds us to build on what students already know, engage students in learning the content, apply active relevant assignments, and help motivate students with assignments that incorporate their current and future interests. We learn (and help our students learn) by accessing new information, actively using that information, and reflecting on our learning (Fink, 2003). Additionally specific technology models will help us as faculty synthesize and build on our own skills as we continue to ask questions and incorporate technologies into our teaching.

Appendixes A and B provide two guides for advancing our work with technologies, (a) our New Technology Readiness Inventory and (b) our

Integrated Learning Triangle for Teaching With Technologies. The readiness inventory provides a checklist approach based on a broad mentoring model (Zachary, 2000) to determine our readiness, opportunities, and motivations for learning about teaching with a particular technology as well as what opportunities and resources are available to us (see Appendix A). Learning a new technology such as Camtasia then might be guided by this checklist of considerations. The checklist helps faculty document opportunities and challenges as well as assess faculty readiness for specific teaching technologies. See the example of how an educator used the checklist in Exhibit 1.2.

Exhibit 1.2

LEARNING A NEW TECHNOLOGY (FIRSTHAND ACCOUNT FROM AN ANONYMOUS AUTHOR)

As a faculty member seeking to enhance my audio presence with online students, I was seeking opportunities for gaining a technology and the know-how to use it. Using the New Technology Readiness Inventory (see Appendix A) I gained some ideas for following up on this need. At our university I found both resources and an initial training session to prepare me to learn the new (to me) Camtasia. I was motivated and ready to learn.

After making a special trip to our college, I arrived early and ready to go. As the session began, I started stressing out because I did not realize the variety of things I could do with the Camtasia technology and thought I had come to the wrong session. Then I calmed down and focused on the parts I wanted. The session helped me confirm that my goal of providing brief audio clips to an online class made sense. I then scheduled a follow-up session with the Camtasia presenter, who had offered further mentoring services. At this follow-up session I got a sense that my planned project was feasible from a technical standpoint. Then I needed to think about how it was doable from a pedagogical standpoint. Here is where I started using the Integrated Learning Triangle for Teaching With Technologies to guide me (see Appendix B).

As I learn Camtasia I am not starting from scratch. I am using teaching skills I have learned throughout my career and have organized around adult education principles. I have created class outlines and I know how to interact with a group of students to engage them in learning. Key points for me to consider beyond the physical how-to of Camtasia now relate much more to pulling educational concepts together. Pushing the big red start button on the technology is the least of my worries. Instead I am focusing on organizing manageable content bites that will encourage students in their own readings and activities. I am thinking about tricky concepts that I could describe in additional content bites. I am thinking about how I can make the information relevant to the students with my examples and theirs.

Gaining comfort with a particular technology, we may then prepare to design an assignment or course using that particular technology. The Integrated Learning Triangle for Teaching With Technologies, influenced by the work of Fink (2003), and based on best practice evidence and theory, provides further direction in planning to use technology in teaching. The three concepts organizing the Integrated Learning Triangle are: objectives/learning goals, beginning assessment/feedback/evaluation, and engaging teaching and learning activities. These concepts are then influenced by a particular setting's logistics, resources, and context.

A set of questions organized around the mnemonic BEBOLDER (Best Evidence, Educational theories, Beginning assessments, Objectives, Logistics, Decisions, Evaluation/Feedback, and Review/Revisions) accompanies the Integrated Learning Triangle and will be referred to in future chapters (see Appendix B). The Integrated Learning Triangle helps faculty document opportunities and challenges for student learning, as well as assess faculty considerations in planning a course, lesson plan, or assignment using technology.

Technology will keep evolving and present us with both challenges and opportunities for being flexible and creative. In new areas, where there is limited research, we have to rely on solid theory, educational principles, and best practices. Gaining a toolkit built around broad teaching principles and concepts helps faculty stay flexible and adapt to change. Case examples throughout the text will help the reader consider opportunities for using the template with varied content. Promoting effective and efficient use of a broad array of technologies, the BEBOLDER template sets the stage for lifelong faculty learning and planning that will promote student learning with technologies.

SUMMARY

This is a book about understanding teaching technologies in partnership with pedagogy. We are being asked to teach in new ways that differ from the ways in which we were taught. New approaches are needed for educating ourselves in using technology as well. Since technology will continue to be a moving target, we need to focus on pedagogy and student learning goals, building the technology around goals to support learning. As technology changes, we can tweak our technology skills and continue to use our educational principles and best practices. As educators reflecting on our practice, we will consider questions for ongoing thought and learning resources with each chapter. Our goal is to share guides for keeping up with teaching technologies without being overwhelmed. Ideas and activities for self-directed learning are incorporated throughout the text.

ENDING REFLECTION

1. What is the most important content that you learned in this chapter?
2. What are your plans for using the information in this chapter in your future teaching endeavors?
3. What are your further learning goals?

GUIDELINES FOR WHAT IT MEANS TO TEACH WITH TECHNOLOGY

Quick Tips for Teaching

1. Orient students to their learning responsibilities and self-directed learning opportunities from the beginning of class.
2. Gain familiarity with Web-based resources designed to support faculty in teaching with technologies such as Quality and Safety Education for Nurses (QSEN) resources.

Questions for Further Reflection

1. What technology resources are you currently using in your teaching?
2. What differences exist in teaching with technologies in the classroom versus teaching about technologies in the clinical setting?
3. What technology resources are easily accessible in your school in addition to those you are currently using? What makes your school unique in technologies for teaching and learning?

Learning Activity: Self-Reflection on Technologies and Pedagogy

As you begin your work in teaching with technologies, consider the following self-assessment, indicating "Agree" or "Disagree" with each of the following statements. As you review further chapters (or discuss the survey with colleagues) see if your opinions change or stay the same.

1. ____ Helping students become self-directed learners takes on increasing importance in teaching with technologies.
2. ____ Active learning has limited relevance for online courses/classes.
3. ____ Technology has made information literacy and searching the literature easier concepts for students to understand.
4. ____ Orientation strategies take up more time than they are worth for high-fidelity patient simulations.
5. ____ Electronic medical records can serve as tools to promote student critical thinking.
6. ____ Student–faculty boundary setting has gotten easier with the advent of Web 2.0 and online social spaces such as Facebook.
7. ____ Students in observer roles can learn with simulation just as well as students with actual case roles.
8. ____ Clickers (audience response systems) in the classroom promote opportunities for gaining test-taking skills.
9. ____ Fall safety projects have little to do with teaching data management.
10. ____ Rubrics, in addition to evaluation, serve as effective student learning tools.
11. ____ Technology provides numerous ways to organize and facilitate student clinical work.
12. ____ Students need opportunities to learn critique of Web-based audiovisuals.

Online Resources for Further Learning

- The TIGER Initiative (Health Information Technology). The TIGER competencies and suggested targets for knowledge, skill, and attitude development during prelicensure education are identified: http://www.tiger summit.com/
- Davis, T., & Murrell, P. (1994). *Turning teaching into learning. The role of student responsibility in the collegiate experience* (ERIC Document Reproduction Service No. ED372702). Retrieved October 16, 2009, from http://www.learn2study.org/teachers/student_resp.htm

■ Quality and Safety Education for Nurses (QSEN) resources. A Robert Wood Johnson Initiative, this project provides interesting tools and resources to promote student learning: http://www.qsen.org

REFERENCES

Carnegie Mellon University. (2009). *Enhancing education: Teaching principles.* Retrieved October 16, 2009, from http://www.cmu.edu/taching/principles/teaching.html

Chickering A. W., & Gamson, A. F. (1987). *Seven principles for good practice in undergraduate education.* Retrieved October 16, 2009, from http://honolulu.hawaii.edu/intranet/committees/FacDevCom/guidebk/teachtip/7princip.htm

Commission on Behavioral and Social Sciences and Education. (1999). *How people learn: Bridging research and practice.* Washington, DC: National Academy Press.

Fink, L. D. (2003). *Creating significant learning experiences: An integrated approach to designing college courses.* San Francisco: Jossey-Bass.

Health and Human Services. (2004). *The decade of health information technology: Delivering consumer-centric and information-rich health care.* Retrieved October 16, 2009, from http://www.hhs.gov/news/press/2004pres/20040721a.html

Institute of Medicine. (2008). *Retooling for an aging America: Building the health care workforce.* Retrieved October 16, 2009, from http://www.iom.edu/CMS/3809/40113/53452.aspx

Knowles, M. (1984). *Andragogy in action: Applying modern principles of adult education.* San Francisco: Jossey-Bass.

Quality and Safety Education for Nurses. (2009). *Home page.* Retrieved October 16, 2009, from http://www.qsen.org/

Skiba, D., Connors, H., & Jeffries, P. (2009). Information technologies and the transformation of nursing education. *Nursing Outlook, 56*(5), 225–230.

Zachary, L. J. (2000). *The mentor's guide: Facilitating effective learning relationships.* San Francisco: Jossey-Bass.

2

Keeping Up With Changing Technology, Self-Directed Learning, and Lifelong Learning

CHAPTER GOAL

Gain practical tips for using self-directed learning and technologies for lifelong learning.

BEGINNING REFLECTION

1. What experiences have you had with self-directed learning (SDL)?
2. What ways do you currently teach or encourage others to use SDL?
3. What ways might technology assist you in your own SDL practices or in guiding your students in SDL?

INTRODUCTION

Clinical knowledge is changing rapidly with the advent of technology. Faculty can no longer hope to convey all clinical information to students in the classroom. At best, faculty can assist students in learning broad concepts and then prepare them to keep up with the changing details. The concepts of SDL and lifelong learning are critical in our technology-rich age. SDL is a tool that all will need to stay current as clinical professionals. Student knowledge gained in our courses will be rapidly out of date if we don't help them acquire skills as self-directed, lifelong learners. While this chapter focuses on helping students use SDL, we can also consider the place of SDL in our own faculty roles, especially as it relates to teaching with technologies.

Interestingly, technologies play a key role in both the need for SDL and in providing opportunities for keeping up. Technology provides opportunities for dealing with the complexity and massive information presented to us daily. As we struggle to find new ways to keep up in a time of information overload, the classics of SDL can prove useful. The skills of SDL will promote ongoing faculty learning needs to help facilitate our students' learning. Technologies play a key role in keeping up with and managing our ongoing learning needs. For both faculty and students the Web makes SDL easier than ever.

While faculty often have comfort with SDL, what will it mean for our students? Faculty will have students for just a short time in classes. It is imperative we teach them SDL skills to maintain a knowledge base as clinicians. In this chapter, strategies for engaging ourselves and our students to become self-directed, lifelong learners are described.

WHAT DO WE MEAN BY SELF-DIRECTED LEARNING?

Knowles (1975) identified a self-directed learner as an adult who seeks to take learning initiative, diagnose learning needs, formulate learning goals, identify learning resources, and choose or implement learning plans and evaluation. SDL as a component of adult education has been documented extensively by Hiemstra and Brockett (1994). A related concept, lifelong learning has been described as a process of learning that depends on individual needs as well as interests and learning skills and that continues throughout one's lifetime (Hiemstra, 2002). For our discussion, lifelong learning is considered a continuation or part of SDL.

Understanding what SDL means to different individuals and building on this meaning provides beginning teaching/learning direction. SDL is not, as the term might suggest, focused on totally independent study and learning. The concept of SDL can be considered from a variety of perspectives and may mean different things to different people. For many classes, SDL will be only one aspect of the course. For example:

- In clinical labs, SDL might mean asking students to prepare independently for a check-off as part of varied clinical assignments.
- In the classroom setting, it may mean choosing a project to complete from a menu of options.
- At a distance education site, it might mean completing self-directed modules via the Web.

The SDL concept has taken on increased relevance with the advent of online learning and the need to coach students at a distance in their learning activities. Assigning beginning students a large textbook and telling them to "know everything" is obviously not the intent of SDL. Hiemstra and Brockett (1994) reported it is important to know that SDL is not an all-or-nothing concept, SDL does not imply learning in isolation, and SDL is not an easy way for faculty to opt out of teaching.

Are SDL and lifelong learning the same thing? The two concepts seem to be quite similar. The authors, for example, have used technology as part of SDL since graduate school when first going to the library to find needed references and then to the copy machine to make copies for further reading. While SDL approaches have changed over the years, the authors believe they gained the basics of identifying a need, a plan, and tools as self-directed learners and have since used these skills as lifelong learners. It seems that SDL and lifelong learning are similar concepts with a time focus built in.

SDL can vary from simple learning choices to creating full independent study courses. For our purposes as educators, the SDL discussion is twofold. First, SDL is considered in helping learners see their role in learning while becoming more accountable for their own learning. Second, SDL involves helping learners enhance their enthusiasm, skill set, and resources for becoming lifelong learners. This second point ties importantly to providing student learning tools or competencies needed by all students, such as information literacy. Without this competency, students will be unable to keep up in using evidence-based practice in their future clinical roles.

SDL includes being proactive in gaining skills for ongoing learning. Fink (2003) speaks to the importance of identifying oneself as a learner and the importance of learning how to learn. Motivating ourselves and our students to be lifelong learners is key. Selected aspects of SDL include the following (Hiemstra & Brockett, 1994):

- SDL includes a sense of appreciating learning skills and valuing learning opportunities.
- SDL has varying degrees, ranging from simple assignment choices to creating objectives and plans for an independent study.
- SDL involves helping students learn to self-assess and identify what they know and what they still need to know (i.e., knowledge gaps) about a specific concept.
- SDL incorporates helping students gain tools, techniques, and resources that support learning and accessing this information for knowledge gaps.
- SDL involves a student–faculty partnership approach to learning and differs from a traditional classroom lecture approach where students may be somewhat passive learners.

As noted, SDL can be considered broadly and varies from those students who are provided some direction and opportunities for assignment choice to those who take primary responsibility for their learning plans. The goal for most courses will be to help students take a more active role and accountability for their learning, so that the graduate accepts responsibility for their own self-directed and lifelong learning.

THEORY BACKGROUND FOR SELF-DIRECTED LEARNING

Adult education and SDL are closely related. Adult education concepts include building on past experiences of the learner, making content relevant, and making content applied and useful for the learner. Consistent with SDL, as students learn about a new respiratory illness for example, they are reminded to build on past coursework and experiences with basic structural and functional concepts of the respiratory system learned in core science courses. Faculty guide students in considering the best resource for gaining the relevant content and then in applying the new information with cases and quizzes that will be relevant to practice.

SDL is not a linear approach to learning, but rather is complex. SDL concepts are consistent with constructivist learning theory, which argues that students construct learning or knowledge gained to fit their contexts (Savery & Duffy, 1995). The individual uses the information and becomes the owner of knowledge. Students are ultimately in control of accepting and incorporating information into their own experiences. For faculty, then, a better understanding of students' past experiences with and current understanding of specific content is key to supporting student learning. Learner assessments can help identify where the gaps or problems are.

LEARNING ASSESSMENTS, BENCHMARKS, AND PLANS FOR SELF-DIRECTED LEARNING

In its most basic form, SDL is based on self-assessments with benchmarks, learning resources, and a plan that helps achieve the learning goals. For faculty as learners, these tools provide a way to consider what we already know, what we still need to know, and strategies for achieving important deficits (a plan for getting there). We as faculty can begin by focusing on our own learning self-assessment, which involves evaluating our current knowledge of our content areas based on accepted benchmarks. Identifying resources and learning plans can then guide us. After gaining this skill set for ourselves, our focus will be how we can best help our students do the same.

The Learning Assessment

Learning assessments provide baseline data for creating our learning plans. To complete a learning assessment, we need to know how to self-assess against a standard. As faculty we will identify standards for our clinical competencies as well as our educator competencies. So we will take stock of our own knowledge deficits, for example, in teaching with technologies. The learning activities presented in this book provide broad approaches to guide faculty reflections related to selected educator topics.

Learning Benchmarks

Benchmarks (consistent with criteria or standards) are basic elements in completing learning assessments. In education, for example, entire books have been written about teacher self-assessment against designated benchmarks, such as a classic work by Bailey (1981). Teaching/learning self-assessment standards or competencies for those teaching clinical courses might also come from sources such as the National League for Nursing. The competencies drafted by this organization serve as a type of benchmark to guide teachers in self-assessing (National League for Nursing, 2005).

Clinical competencies will be important to faculty as well. The benchmarks for self-assessment may include using informal educational systems such as those provided by national professional organizations and health care associations. Those seeking standards for addressing clinical competencies such as geriatrics might seek standards provided by national geriatric organizations such as the American Geriatrics Society. Those seeking to gain and document expertise in palliative care, for example, go to professional organizations' standards and create an assessment and learning plan for themselves. Our benchmarks depend on our current role focus and accepted standards at a point in time. See a sample guide for learning assessment in this chapter's "Learning Activity" section.

Learning Plan

In part, this book will help us as faculty be self-directed in designing our own teaching with technology plans and learning tasks. This book provides concepts that are important to consider in our teaching. The New Technology Readiness Inventory (Appendix A), for example, is available to assess your resources, opportunities, and support for learning a new technology. Readers decide the topics for their projects and activities. The Integrated Learning Triangle for Teaching With Technologies (Appendix B) serves as a tool for further planning your teaching approaches. For example, if you want to learn more to help you make changes in a physical assessment course (whether online or in the classroom) you could use physical assessment as the background or context for a majority of your thinking as you read this text. You will be guided to think about how (or if) technologies would help achieve learning goals. You can create a package of experiences that are relevant for your teaching/learning needs. Student contracts can help students better understand their responsibility in learning. Further details on using learning contracts as a form of SDL are provided in a detailed 12-step model by Hiemstra (2005).

FACULTY ROLE, HELPING STUDENTS BECOME SELF-DIRECTED LEARNERS

Being a Coach

Teaching toward ongoing lifelong learning requires faculty to take on new roles, including coaching or facilitating student learning. Faculty transition from a more traditional lecturer role to emphasize building teaching/learning partnerships with students. A coaching role in working with students provides opportunity to help students frame and focus important course concepts. Consistent with the coach analogy, faculty support students in their individual learning but also bring them together as a learning team.

We can help students identify knowledge needs and assist students to identify learning tasks and selected approaches to gain requisite knowledge. Assessing and planning for learning applies to our students as well. Faculty do more than pass on information; they provide resources and rubrics to guide expected outcomes. Our faculty role with teaching technologies involves helping students understand what they need to know and how to access that information. Faculty provide opportunities for students to gain new information and do something with this information in the form of assignments. Faculty coach or facilitate, helping students move forward, assisting them and providing the resources they need.

The idea is to encourage and provide student assignments that help students learn about concepts in engaging ways. In a nursing course, it can often mean that the instructor guides individual learning by providing specific active learning assignments or providing a menu of activities or assignments (designed to achieve course outcomes) from which students choose those they find most relevant and meaningful.

In a face-to-face class, faculty might provide assignments that engage students in viewing a specific health care organization, such as the online Alzheimer's Association. Students have an opportunity to actively review a Web site and seek evidence-based resources they can use with current and future patients. Once students are aware of this resource, they have access to the information well after they have left a course. They are able to transfer their learning from the classroom to their clinical work.

As noted, a faculty facilitator or coach role in SDL is very different from just handing someone a book, telling them to learn the information, and then providing a test. Orientation to learning, student reflective self-assessments, and motivational strategies are important concepts in our toolkit and apply to many aspects of teaching and learning.

Orientating Students to Self-Directed Learning

An orientation can provide a framework for student learning in a course. This orientation includes not only learning about or previewing course activities, but orienting to the various learning tools, assignment plans, and testing plans that will be used. As noted by Fink (2003), students should understand why and how these tools are important in helping them learn their profession.

A good orientation frames the class, providing students with guides as to what they will be learning, what the course process will be, and what course outcomes and expectations of what should happen will be. Orientation includes helping students identify the best learning resources available for their role as self-directed learners, including course tools such as textbooks. A one-page class organizer may be provided that synthesizes and gives direction as to what the course is about and how it will proceed. Orientation frameworks can provide students with further ideas for their own learning plans.

In a study that surveyed students about their perceptions of high-fidelity simulation experiences (Conejo, 2009), for example, students reported wanting orientation information that answered the following questions: What is the main theme of the lab? What is expected of us? What skills do we need? Where are things? How do things work? Will we have an actual patient chart? What are the rules? Is this for learning or testing? Providing a good orientation allows students to prepare and understand their role as partners in learning.

An evidence-based review abstract, "Online Readiness to Learn," is shared at the end of the chapter. This systematic review provides faculty direction for developing orientation programs using online learning courses and student readiness to learn as an exemplar.

Guiding Students via Reflective Self-Assessments

Reflective self-assessments are important tools in SDL, providing students one way to consider what they know and don't know and what they need to further learn. Fink (2003) noted that one relatively easy way to both engage students and extend learning includes asking our students to complete self-reflections. Reflection provides the opportunity for students to integrate new information into their own experiences. Reflection, an active process in which students consider their experiences, helps students think about what they are learning. While this has been noted as particularly relevant in online courses, it has relevance across all types of classes and technologies for better preparing our students.

Reflective exercises add an active component to learning and provide an opportunity for students to synthesize and share their experiences with others and to further cement learning. Fink (2003) noted that significant learning is enhanced as students reflect on their activities. Reflection can enhance self-evaluation skill as students build on previous experiences and reflect on how an assignment contributed to their learning.

Self-assessments are a form of reflection and are a good place to start an educational endeavor. Performing self-assessments based on a standard can help students gain skills in judging the quality of their work; they judge their self-knowledge and determine when more learning is needed.

Self-assessments help determine what has been learned and what still needs to be achieved. To self-assess, students need criterion or standards to measure their learning against. The key points are to help students know the most respected standard and reference sources. Rubrics that summarize key points for learning (pre- and postclass) provide students' guides. Additionally, portfolios provide a way to record reflections over a course of time.

A variety of technologies from clickers (automated response systems) to online surveys provide simple tools with preclass questions that can provide faculty with their students' background information on the topic. Asking students to reflect and share experiences about the concept to be discussed is a type of self-assessment.

Learning style assessments are another aspect of self-assessment, helping students recognize their learning styles and how best to set up study plans that match their styles. As students look at their learning styles, they can determine if they are visual learners, auditory learners, hands-on learners, or some mix. For example, recognizing they are visual learners and can learn/recall information best that is visually displayed can promote successful student planning (Fleming, 2009). Gaining this information can help students identify best strategies and begin learning plans. Exhibit 2.1 provides examples of learning styles inventories that students can complete.

Exhibit 2.1

LEARNING STYLE ASSESSMENTS FOR BEGINNING SDL

Use the following resources to help students gain familiarity with their learning styles:

■ How do I learn best? Complete the VARK assessment for a determination of your learning style: http://www.vark-learn.com/english/page.asp?p=questionnaire

■ How can I build study skills based on my learning style? After completing the VARK assessment, refer to the VARK Help Sheets specific to your learning styles to gain ideas for your learning plans: http://www.vark-learn.com/english/page.asp?p=helpsheets

---

Motivating Students Toward Self-Directed Learning

Students learn more if they care about what they are learning. Svinicki (2005) notes that goal orientation is situation specific. Consistent with adult education and authentic learning, striving to keep learning interesting and relevant relates to student motivation. Whether in a class, a course, or a program, it helps to begin by thinking about how we get our students to care and be enthused about the topic as well as ready to join class conversations. A son's physical therapy assistant (PTA) program provides an example. The summer before the PTA program started, he received a very upbeat letter introducing him to the program and school. Before school started, he was a student member in the national professional organization and knew what kinds of things he would be doing his first weeks in class. This was a highly motivated young man who headed off to school.

Providing learning activity choices is consistent with adult education theory, helping make assignments more relevant to students' needs and interests.

Learning activity choices promote autonomy and motivation (Hofer, 2006). The importance of building on intrinsic motivation and expectancy of success is also noted by Svinicki (2005). She describes concepts ranging from meaningful learning activities to choice in assignments to promote goal orientation and to create an attitude of learning mastery and expectancy of success (see further examples of promoting a success orientation to learning, Exhibit 2.2). Students might, for example, create teaching pamphlets for clinical patients or develop study resources to share with peers on topics that have immediate relevance for them. Problem-

Exhibit 2.2

ENCOURAGE A SUCCESS ORIENTATION TO LEARNING

- Develop assignments based on knowledge and skills that are important to learn.
- Create learning tasks for students that just exceed an anticipated base capability but that are still within their reach; expect them to succeed.
- Encourage the building of a community of learners in your class, where everyone supports everyone else's attempts to learn.
- Make the classroom a safe place for learning, responding to students' attempts to learn in a caring way.
- If possible, give the learners some choices in what or the way they learn (learning assignments).
- Be a good model of a success-oriented learner in your own scholarship.

Influenced by Svinicki (2005).

---

solving assignments serve as motivators in increasing student curiosity. Creative teaching strategies that highlight a variety of authentic activities can motivate active learning in health profession courses (Herrman, 2008).

Building SDL into the "what next?" aspect of learning, Fink (2003) describes the importance of helping students set further learning goals. Motivation comes as a function of goals and expectations, so it benefits students to set learning goals and evaluate for progress periodically or at the end of a course (Hofer, 2006). Encouraging students to take owner-ship of their learning outcomes or consider who the learning belongs to (Walvoord & Anderson, 1998) helps avoid an us/them dichotomy that can develop with teacher-controlled grades. Helping students consider how they can partner with faculty to enhance their learning is a goal of SDL.

Self-Directed Learning, Technology, and Enrichment or Remediation

Additionally, technology provides opportunities for using SDL in student enrichment or remediation. A good example of SDL and technology is student use of computers for practice testing. Computer-based practice testing provides students with ongoing learning opportunities rather than just testing. Online testing programs such as Assessment Technologies Institute (ATI) and Kaplan provide opportunities for students' SDL. Students, if properly oriented, can see benefits of knowing where their weaknesses are and what learning areas they need to focus on. This is very different than testing where students are simply seeking a grade and are not aware of the areas in which they are performing well or poorly. Judicious use of automated practice tests can provide students with immediate feedback on individual answers and broader individualized learning plans with areas of study outlined.

As discussed previously in the chapter, the evidence-based review abstract "Online Readiness to Learn" is provided in Exhibit 2.3. This synthesis of best evidence provides further direction for our work as educators.

Exhibit 2.3

EVIDENCE-BASED REVIEW ABSTRACT: ONLINE READINESS TO LEARN

Compiled by: Jamie S. Myers, RN, MN, AOCN

Online education is becoming ever more prevalent across a variety of degree programs and other venues for nursing education, such as staff development and continuing education. Not all nurses are computer savvy, and many express frustrations related to lack of expertise. Identification of best practices for online education is important to the nursing community, as is the assessment of nurses' readiness to learn in the online environment.

A systematic literature review was performed to explore the teaching/learning concept of online readiness to learn. PubMed, CINAHL, and ERIC databases were searched for the following broad terms: readiness to learn; e-learning readiness; Web-based learning readiness; online readiness; orientation for staff development; online learning; and Web-based learning. References published in 2000 or later were accepted. Search results were summarized in an annotated bibliography with two primary themes emerging: technological and behavioral readiness to learn. Technological readiness involves learners' skill and competence with computers; access to sufficient hardware, software, and the Internet; and administrative support of dedicated time for online education.

Behavioral readiness is dependent on a number of concepts such as self-directedness, motivation, self-discipline, and autonomy. These characteristics were reported to be necessary for success with online learning. Strong recommendations were made for both technological and behavioral readiness assessment prior to initiating online coursework. Information gleaned from the systematic literature review was used to design a model case. Using concepts of self-directed learning and based on adult education principles, a program to promote success in the online learning environment for registered nurses pursuing a bachelor's degree in nursing was suggested. Based on the literature, a number of active learning components were included to engage the learner. Participants would be asked to complete the following self-directed activities: download assigned readings from a specific Web site, utilize a Web link to a program to conduct a self-assessment of their particular learning style (i.e., visual, auditory, kinesthetic), complete a self-

(Continued)

Exhibit 2.3

EVIDENCE-BASED REVIEW ABSTRACT: ONLINE READINESS TO LEARN (*Continued*)

reflection paper describing personal strengths and opportunities for growth in online learning skills, and participate in the online discussion board to share concrete plans for enhancing the skills necessary for online learning. Grading rubrics are suggested to evaluate achievements. Future research could explore the relation of these strategies to increased online program completion.

Bibliography

Atak, L. (2002). A descriptive study of registered nurses' experiences with Web-based learning. *Journal of Advanced Nursing, 40*, 457–465.

Atak, L. (2003). Becoming a Web-based learner: Registered nurses' experiences. *Journal of Advanced Nursing, 44*, 289–297.

Clarke, A., Lewis, D., Cole, I., & Ringrose, L. (2005). A strategic approach to developing e-learning capability for healthcare. *Health Information and Libraries Journal, 22*(Suppl. 2), 33–41.

Cobb, S. C. (2004). Internet continuing education for health care professionals: An integrative review. *The Journal of Continuing Education in the Health Care Professions, 24*, 171–180.

Curran-Smith, J., & Best, S. (2004). An experience with an on-line learning environment to support a change in practice in an emergency department. *CIN: Computers Informatics Nursing, 22*(2), 107–110.

Lee, J., Hong, N. L., & Ling, N. L. (2002). An analysis of students' preparation for the virtual learning environment. *Internet and Higher Education, 4*, 231–242.

MacFadden, R. J. (2005). Souls on ice: Incorporating emotion in Web-based education. *Journal of Technology in Human Services, 23*(1/2), 79–98.

O'Shea, E. (2003). Self-directed learning in nurse education: A review of the literature. *Issues and Innovations in Nursing Education, 43*(1), 62–70.

Phillips, J. M. (2005). Strategies for active learning in online continuing education. *Journal of Continuing Education in Nursing, 36*, 77–83.

Pillay, H., Irving, K., & Tones, M. (2007). Validation of the diagnostic tool for assessing tertiary students' readiness for online learning. *Higher Education Research and Development, 26*, 217–234.

Pullen, D. L. (2006). An evaluative case study of online learning for healthcare professionals. *Journal of Continuing Education in Nursing, 37*, 225–232.

Smith, P. J. (2005). Learning preferences and readiness for online learning. *Educational Psychology, 25*(1), 3–12.

Smith, P. J., Murphy, K. L., & Mahoney, S. E. (2003). Towards identifying factors underlying readiness for online learning: An exploratory study. *Distance Education, 24*, 57–67.

Stokes, C. W., Cannavina, C., & Cannavina, G. (2004). The state of readiness of student health professionals for Web-based learning environments. *Health Informatics Journal, 10*, 195–204

Wilkinson, A., Forbes, A., Bloomfield, J., & Gee, C. F. (2004). An exploration of four Web-based open and flexible learning modules in post-registration nurse education. *International Journal of Nursing Studies, 41*, 411–424.

SUMMARY

The concepts of SDL and lifelong learning are closely linked and will become increasingly important for students and faculty in our rapidly changing clinical worlds. Technology resources provide opportunities to enhance our faculty roles in both using and teaching SDL for lifelong learning. Teaching tools such as orientations, reflective self-assessments, and assignments that help motivate students provide initial direction. To keep up with the evidence base of the future and continue to provide quality care to our patients, SDL is a needed skill.

ENDING REFLECTION

1. What is the most important content that you learned in this chapter?
2. What are your plans for using the information in this chapter in your future teaching endeavors?
3. What are your further learning goals?

GUIDELINES FOR KEEPING UP WITH CHANGING TECHNOLOGY, SELF-DIRECTED LEARNING, AND LIFELONG LEARNING

Quick Tips to Promote Self-Directed Learning

1. Provide orientation guides at the beginning of a course. Include orientation to textbooks and technology resources (highlighting key features of each) as well as course content.
2. Have students complete self-assessments on study and learning skills from online resources and set further learning goals.
3. Provide online calendars with assignment dates and encourage students to plot out their study times.
4. When possible, provide students with an opportunity to choose an assignment from a brief list of options that all meet objectives.

Questions for Further Reflection

1. When does adult education start?
2. When (or at what level) is the best time to introduce concepts of SDL to students?

3. Is there a component of group learning or sharing that adds value when using SDL?

Learning Activity: Self-Assessment

How would you rate yourself on the following (low, medium, or high)?

1. I can describe the current role of technologies in my teaching.
2. I have a good basics technology toolkit.
3. I have interest in increasing my technology toolkit.
4. I can name theories that guide my teaching with technology.
5. I am comfortable blending my current teaching strategies with a new blending of technologies.
6. I am confident in my skills as a self-directed learner.

Based on your rating, what initial plan will you generate for your own SDL? How will you use the New Technology Readiness Inventory (Appendix A) and the Integrated Learning Triangle (Appendix B) to assist in your planning?

Online Resources for Further Learning

- Davis, T., & Murrell, P. (1994). *Turning teaching into learning. The role of student responsibility in the collegiate experience* (ERIC Document Reproduction Service No. ED372702): http://www.learn2study.org/teachers/student_resp.htm
- Quality and Safety Education for Nurses (QSEN) resources. A Robert Wood Johnson Initiative, this project provides interesting tools and resources to promote student learning: http://www.qsen.org
- The Technology Informatics Guiding Education Reform (TIGER) Initiative. The TIGER competencies suggest targets for knowledge, skill, and attitude development during prelicensure education: http://www.tigersummit.com/

REFERENCES

Bailey, G. (1981). *Teacher self-assessment, a means for improving classroom instruction.* Washington, DC: National Education Association.

Conejo, P. (2009). *Faculty and student perceptions of preparation for and implementation of high fidelity simulation experiences in associate degree nursing programs.* Unpublished doctoral dissertation, University of Kansas.

Fink, L. D. (2003). *Creating significant learning experiences: An integrated approach to designing college courses.* San Francisco: Jossey-Bass.

Fleming, N. (2009). *VARK, a guide to learning styles.* Retrieved October 16, 2009, from http://www.vark-learn.com/english/index.asp

Herrman, J. (2008). *Creative teaching strategies for the nurse educator.* Philadelphia, PA: FA Davis.

Hiemstra, R. (2002). *Lifelong learning: An exploration of adult and continuing education within a setting of lifelong learning needs* (3rd ed.). Fayetteville, NY: HiTree Press.

Hiemstra, R. (2005). *Techniques, tools, and resources for the self-directed learner.* Retrieved October 16, 2009, from http://www-distance.syr.edu/sdltools.html

Hiemstra, R., & Brockett, R. (1994). *Overcoming resistance to self-direction in adult learning: New directions for adult and continuing education.* San Francisco, CA: Jossey-Bass.

Hofer, B. (2006). Motivation in the college classroom. In W. McKeachie & M. Svinicki (Eds.), *McKeachie's teaching tips: Strategies, research, and theory for college and university teachers* (12th ed., pp. 140–149). Boston, MA: Houghton Mifflin.

Knowles, M. S. (1975). *Self-directed learning. A guide for learners and teachers,* Englewood Cliffs, NJ: Prentice Hall.

National League for Nursing. (2005). *Core competencies of nurse educators with task statements.* Retrieved October 16, 2009, from http://www.nln.org/profdev/pdf/corecompetencies.pdf

Savery, J., & Duffy, T. (1995). Problem based learning: An instructional model and its constructivist framework. *Educational Technology, 35,* 31–38.

Svinicki, M. (2005). *Student goal orientation, motivation, and learning.* Retrieved October 16, 2009, from http://www.theideacenter.org/sites/default/files/Idea_Paper_41.pdf

Walvoord, B., & Anderson, V. (1998). *Effective grading: A tool for learning and assessment.* San Francisco: Jossey-Bass.

3 Theory and Teaching Technologies

CHAPTER GOAL

Recognize the relationship between theories and best practices and their combined impact on both quality teaching with technologies and quality health care.

BEGINNING REFLECTION

1. What are your experiences using theories?
2. What education-related theories do you currently use?
3. What is your familiarity with best practices in education and clinical practice?
4. What do you know about the Institute of Medicine (IOM) reports on quality health care?

INTRODUCTION

Theory is key in guiding teaching with technology. At a time when it is hard to keep up with rapidly changing technology, theories provide direction for teaching and learning. Time-tested classics such as adult education theory meld well with today's technology-rich environment. Theories and models serve as guides in organizing teaching and learning. They can guide our thinking and help us name more easily what we are doing. They can provide consistency or stability for faculty as they move forward with new content or new technologies.

The fairly constant foundation of educational theories stands in the face of constantly changing technology. This stability is encouraging because, while the content being taught and the technologies used to teach will be constantly changing, the theoretical underpinnings of how to teach and why to teach that way will generally not change quickly or dramatically.

Consider, for example, the question of how to teach range of motion. We know that, based on learning theories, the learning process will be facilitated by the students' active participation in the process. It does not matter if they participate in person, through a computer program, or via a virtual game; as long as they are actively involved, students will likely learn more quickly and better remember what they have learned. So the basic theoretical principle of active participation by the learners is unchanged no matter what latest technologies are used to teach students range of motion.

Best teaching and learning practices are guided by theory. In this respect, theories serve several purposes: they provide a structure or framework for teaching activities, they provide an explanation for why content is taught the way it is taught, and they often raise questions or identify issues that, without the framework, might be completely missed or ignored. Whether acknowledged or not, theories help us teach well.

THEORIES: WHAT THEY ARE AND WHAT THEY ARE NOT

Theory refers to the structuring of ideas in creative and rigorous ways to "project a tentative, purposeful, and systematic view of phenomena" (Chinn & Kramer, 2004, p. 51). In our case, if we insert the word *teaching* or *learning* in place of the word *phenomena,* we see that theories provide a means of structuring ideas about teaching (or learning) in a systematic way. Well-developed theories tell us what to do and why to do it.

The application of theories to explain and justify actions is a hallmark of a profession. As educators we use not only teaching/learning theories but a variety of other theories (e.g., motivational theories, change theories, team theories, and developmental theories) as well. Just as important as the structure they provide, theories provide a comprehensive perspective that not only makes questions and concerns more obvious but also provides a context in which to address them.

As with many topics, any discussion of theory is fraught with issues of semantics. What, for example, is the difference between teaching theories, learning theories, and educational theories? While there may be legitimate nuances to the connoisseur, in this book we are more concerned about the practicality of theories in supporting teaching endeavors. For example, the teaching process is facilitated by motivation among students, suggesting that teaching/learning theories alone are not enough. Rather, teaching is enhanced by the simultaneous use of motivational—and other—theories as well.

There are many classic teaching/learning theories that provide the theoretical basis of most educational texts. A brief background can be gained by considering the following classics, which are referenced frequently in the literature (e.g., Kaufman, 2003):

- Behaviorists believe that all behavior is learned through a fairly passive process of conditioning. Knowledge and skills that receive positive rewards are likely acquired, and those that receive negative reinforcement are likely rejected.
- Social learning theory suggests that the learning process consists of interactions between learners, their environment, and the desired knowledge and/or behavior. Observing others in the desired behavior may provide an environmental motivation to learn the behavior. It may also help the learner see the importance of the new knowledge, which may provide the motivation necessary to learn the behavior.
- Humanistic learning theory assumes that each person is a unique individual who deserves respect, freedom, and worth, and has the desire to grow. It emphasizes individual rights, creativity, and spontaneity, and suggests that learning is driven by people's subjective needs.

Three theories in particular provide many of the basic tenants of good teaching with technologies today. A brief summary of each is provided with additional recommended readings. These three theories are adult learning theory, constructivist theory, and complexity theory.

Adult Learning Theory

Referred to as *andragogy* (versus *pedagogy*, which refers to the education of children, but is often used as the more common umbrella term), adult education theory is based largely on the work of Knowles (1980). Adult learners are self-directed, practical, and build on past experience. Their motivation generally has an internal source. They need their life experiences and accumulated knowledge base to be acknowledged, respected, and used. They learn best when they see the immediate relevance and practical application of what they are learning. Many adult learners juggle multiple responsibilities, which can create barriers to education, such as lack of time and money, scheduling problems, and child care issues. Despite these barriers, adult learners are motivated by opportunities for personal advancement, social relationships, and a general desire for their own growth. Adult education theory reminds faculty to build on students' previous learning, engage students with the content, and use active, relevant assignments.

Constructivism

Constructivism emerged from cognitive learning theory and also recognizes the past knowledge and experience of learners. In this theory, learners use that prior knowledge and experience to actively build new knowledge. A pervasive tenet of constructivism is the active nature of learning, from creating the learning environment to participating in learning activities and interacting with peers and faculty. This theory emphasizes the active and autonomous role of students and defines the role of faculty in terms of facilitating that active learning process. Constructivism reminds faculty that students construct their own understandings of concepts based on the content resources and tools we provide them (Savery & Duffy, 1995).

Complexity

Complexity theory provides a way to consider teaching and learning from a nonlinear perspective. Complexity theory has been described as the opposite of chaos theory, focusing on an entire system and its interconnections rather than individual units (Zimmerman, Plsek, & Lindberg, 2008). Since nursing education requires complex learning and takes place in complex clinical situations, this theory is often relevant to our teaching and learning considerations as well.

All theories come with basic assumptions. These assumptions typically lay the groundwork for how concepts are defined and how the theory's concepts relate. Recognizing the assumptions of different theories provides direction in determining which theories best fit a given situation and purpose. A clinical lab on teaching dressing changes provides an example with adult learning theory as an organizing approach. With adult education theory, faculty are reminded to build on students' current levels of information (based on assessment), provide relevant information specific to students' learning needs, and provide an active assignment that engages students in practicing dressing changes. Practical application of teaching and learning theories promotes improved classes.

BEST TEACHING PRACTICES

Like theories, best practices transcend both the content being taught and the technology being used to teach it. So, while there may be several ways to teach safe medication administration (on a classmate, on a patient, or on a computer-generated patient), the same basic theoretical principles and the same basic best practices apply to all methods. This fairly constant foundation of theories and best practices is encouraging. While the content being taught and the technologies used to teach will constantly change, the theoretical underpinnings and best practices regarding how to teach and why to teach that way will generally not change quickly or dramatically.

Best practices are documented strategies, supported by evidence, that produce good teaching and learning outcomes (Billings & Connors, 2009). Twenty years ago Chickering and Gamson (1987) were early best practice adopters, using research to identify seven principles of good teaching and learning in undergraduate education. These practices are noted in Exhibit 3.1.

Exhibit 3.1

BEST PRACTICES: CHICKERING AND GAMSON'S (1987) SEVEN PRINCIPLES OF GOOD TEACHING AND LEARNING IN UNDERGRADUATE EDUCATION

1. Faculty and students need to communicate frequently.
2. Encourage positive relationships among students.
3. Keep the learning process active.
4. Provide feedback promptly and encourage students to self-reflect on their own performance.
5. The time spent on a given topic or task is important.
6. Inform students of high-quality work expectations.
7. Respect students' diverse strengths and learning styles.

Carnegie Mellon University (2009a) has since expanded best teaching principles, which have been developed from a variety of disciplines, using the best evidence available. The teaching principles are:

1. Information gathered about your learners should be used to design the course and teaching strategies.
2. Learning objectives, learning activities, and evaluation must be consistent.
3. Learning outcomes and policy expectations must be explicit.
4. The knowledge and skills to be taught should be prioritized.
5. Faculty should acknowledge and address their own blind spots.
6. Faculty should assume roles that support the students' learning goals.
7. Feedback and reflection should be used to continually revise courses.

The development of best teaching practices from Chickering and Gamson (1987) to Carnegie Mellon University (2009a) suggests that best practices are not entirely static. For example, Chickering and Gamson emphasized time on task (or the amount of time spent on a task), yet it is now recognized that time on task alone is not sufficient for good teaching and learning. In the Carnegie Mellon best practices, engagement, rather than time, is emphasized. Faculty should be aware of this growing body of evidence, and be prepared to draw on and contribute to this evidence.

Learning principles remind us of the important focus on learning as well as teaching, so the students' role as learners must be recognized. Learning principles have also been developed to guide teaching and learning considerations (Carnegie Mellon University, 2009b). These learning principles include:

1. Previous knowledge and experience can either help or hurt future learning.
2. Motivation creates and sustains positive learning behaviors.
3. The way learners organize knowledge affects their appropriate use of that knowledge.
4. Skills and knowledge, synthesis, and application are all necessary for content mastery.
5. Learning requires practice focused on specific goals, as well as focused feedback.

6. Self-directed learners can monitor, evaluate, and adjust their learning activities as needed.
7. Because learners are holistic beings, the social and emotional aspects of the classroom affect their learning.

An evidence-based review abstract, "Learning to Learn With Concept Mapping," is shared at the end of the chapter. Recognizing concepts as the principal components of theories, this systematic review explicitly combines both theory and best practices and provides faculty direction for engaging students in their own learning with orientation sessions on concept mapping.

THEORY, INSTITUTE OF MEDICINE, AND HEALTH PROFESSIONALS IMPLICATIONS

Theories also help organize the vast amounts of information that exist in the rapidly changing clinical world. While this book focuses primarily on theory as a way to organize teaching activities, it is important to recognize that models and theories are useful organizers for clinical content, too. Randomly scattered bits of clinical information are of limited use to students and clinicians. Pulling these information bits together with a conceptual model or theory promotes an organized approach to learning and later recall of the topic. Models of pain management that address structural and functional pathophysiology and then relate it to best pain management evidence are examples.

Knowing and using theories and best teaching practices is vital, but theory without the proper content is useless. It is easy in nursing to become complacent about that content, as there always seems to be too much content and too little time available to teach it. Similarly, it seems as if there is always so much new content to include, yet no old content to relinquish. Using a conceptual (i.e., theoretical) approach to teaching can help faculty make the difficult decisions about what really needs to be taught.

Like the constantly changing teaching technologies that are the focus of this book, technology is creating fast-paced, constant change in the content of clinical practice as well. Consequently, technology affects the content of the clinical content taught to future health care clinicians. The IOM has published a series of reports (see Exhibit 3.2) on varying aspects of the health care system, with the intent of improving that very system. The number and extent of these reports indicate the need for faculty and students alike to understand and apply the principles promulgated. Further discussion regarding the import of these reports for nursing education is provided by Finkelman and Kenner (2009). Technology provides a powerful tool with which to collect, analyze, and disseminate the evidence necessary to establish these best clinical recommendations.

Exhibit 3.2

IMPORTANT IOM REPORTS SPECIFIC TO CLINICAL HEALTH PROFESSIONS EDUCATION

Each of these reports can be located online by running an Internet search for the title. A summary of the reports is provided by Finkelman and Kenner (2009).

Safety Reports:

To Err Is Human (1999)
Patient Safety: Achieving a New Standard of Care (2004)

Quality Reports:

Crossing the Quality Chasm (2001)
Envisioning the National Healthcare Quality (2001)
Priority Areas for National Action: Transforming Healthcare Quality (2003)

Leadership Report:

Leadership by Example: Coordinating Government Roles in Improving Healthcare Quality (2003)

Public Health Reports:

The Future of the Public's Health in the 21st Century (2003)
Who Will Keep the Public Health? (2003)
Unequal Treatment: Confronting Racial and Ethnic Disparities in Healthcare (2002)
Guidance for the National Healthcare Disparities Report (2002)

Nursing Report:

Keeping Patients Safe: Transforming the Work Environment for Nurses (2004)

Health Professions Education Report:

Health Professional Education: A Bridge to Quality (2003)

The IOM reports (Finkelman & Kenner, 2009) have identified 20 priority areas of care for evidence-based clinical practice. To ensure that clinicians are properly prepared to address these priority areas and the systems in which they work, critical curricular components are also identified. Six improvement goals relate to health care being safe, effective, patient-centered, timely, efficient, and equitable (IOM, 2001).

These IOM recommendations are comprehensive and far reaching. The reports demonstrate the extent to which the entire context in which health care providers, and nurses in particular, are educated must change in order to accomplish these goals. Educational implications of the IOM resources have been further discussed (Finkelman & Kenner, 2009). Technology represents a key mechanism by which best clinical practices are established and best teaching practices facilitate their implementation through the education of both new and established practitioners. Five core competencies for health professions have been identified and their acknowledgement has been widespread. The broad concepts provide direction as well, for teaching with technologies. The five core competencies identified by the IOM (2003) include the following:

- Provide patient-centered care.
- Work in interdisciplinary teams.
- Employ evidence-based practice.
- Apply quality improvement.
- Utilize informatics.

TRIANGLE OF INTEGRATED LEARNING FOR TEACHING WITH TECHNOLOGIES

In the Triangle of Integrated Learning (Appendix B), both theories and best teaching practices are represented by the outer circle. They are part of the broader sphere in which a specific teaching activity is situated. Theories and best practices represent knowledge that is foundational to educational experiences in general, and so they are represented by the outside circle in which any particular teaching activity and related decisions are placed.

As discussed previously in the chapter, the evidence-based review abstract "Learning to Learn With Concept Mapping" is provided in Exhibit 3.3. This synthesis of best evidence provides further direction for our work as educators.

Exhibit 3.3

EVIDENCE-BASED REVIEW ABSTRACT: LEARNING TO LEARN WITH CONCEPT MAPPING

Compiled by: Patricia Conejo, MSN, RN, WHNP

Students need to be prepared as lifelong learners. Helping students learn to use concept maps is one strategy to promote critical thinking and lifelong learning. Literature supports that these holistic visual representations encourage active learning, improve critical thinking, and increase knowledge retention; students better understand patient conditions and plan nursing care. Fink (2003) described the importance of helping students learn to learn with the tools we provide. Strategies for teaching students how best to learn with concept maps (including literature on best evidence for concept maps and guidelines for helping students learn with concept maps) were reviewed.

Recommendations for best practices drawn from the literature included providing clear instructions, using a valid and reliable rubric, and creating opportunities for reflection via peer and faculty feedback. Piloting of the best evidence with a group of students included a narrated PowerPoint presentation on Learning to Learn with Concept Maps, assignment guidelines, a feedback worksheet, and a rubric. The assignment was to draw a concept map for one of two situations of relevance for nursing students, organization of the multiple course assignments for the semester or time management to balance the demands of work, home, and school. Student responses, including students' concept maps, written feedback, and in-class discussion, were evaluated for themes and evidence of critical thinking.

A major theme that emerged was student openness to trying concept mapping, but not being accustomed to the non-linear approach. The greatest challenge appeared to lie in motivating students to take the time to reorient their thinking patterns to this more holistic, big picture approach. Further study of effective methods for moving students in this direction is needed. Students who develop their high-level thinking skills as a result of concept mapping will be better prepared for ongoing learning and to care for patients in the increasingly complex and rapidly evolving environment of today's health care.

Bibliography

Ausubel, D. P. (1960). The use of advance organizers in the learning and retention of meaningful, verbal material. *Journal of Educational Psychology, 51*, 267–272.

Billings, D. M., & Halstead, J. A. (2006). *Teaching in nursing: A guide for faculty* (2nd ed.). St. Louis, MO: Elsevier.

Facione, P. A., & Facione, N. C. (1994). *Holistic critical thinking scoring rubric.* Millbrae, CA: The California Academic Press.

Fink, L. D. (2003). *Creating significant learning experiences: An integrated approach to designing college courses.* San Francisco: Jossey-Bass.

Finkelman, A., & Kenner, C. (2009). *Teaching IOM: Implications of the Institute of Medicine Reports for nursing education* (2nd ed.). Silver Spring, MD: American Nurses Association.

(Continued)

Exhibit 3.3

EVIDENCE-BASED REVIEW ABSTRACT: LEARNING TO LEARN WITH CONCEPT MAPPING (*Continued*)

Fonteyn, M. (2007). Concept mapping: An easy teaching strategy that contributes to understanding and may improve critical thinking. *Journal of Nursing Education, 46*, 199–200.

Hicks-Moore, S. L., & Pastrik, P. J. (2006). Evaluating critical thinking in clinical concept maps: A pilot study. *International Journal of Nursing Education Scholarship, 3*, 1–15.

Kostovich, C. T., Poradzisz, M., Wood, K., & O'Brien, K. L. (2007). Learning style preference and student aptitude for concept maps. *Journal of Nursing Education, 46*, 225–231.

Moni, R. W., Beswick, E., & Moni, K. B. (2005). Using student feedback to construct a scoring rubric for a concept map in physiology. *Advances in Physiology Education, 29*, 197–203.

Schuster, P. M. (2002). *Concept mapping: A critical-thinking approach to care planning.* Philadelphia: F.A. Davis.

Taylor, J., & Wros, P. (2007). Concept mapping: A nursing model for care planning. *Journal of Nursing Education, 46*, 211–215.

SUMMARY

As faculty struggle to keep up with rapidly changing content and technologies, theories and models serve as tools to help organize approaches and provide consistency and stability. Supported by the available evidence, these theories and best teaching practices provide the guidance necessary to make teaching endeavors successful. The IOM calls for a similar process in the health care system, in which best clinical practices would provide the guidance necessary for good clinical outcomes. As these best clinical practices emerge, technologies provide teaching platforms for disseminating information to students and health care providers.

ENDING REFLECTION

1. What is the most important content that you learned in this chapter?
2. What are your plans for using the information in this chapter in your future teaching endeavors?
3. What are your further learning goals?

GUIDELINES FOR THEORY AND TEACHING TECHNOLOGIES

Quick Tips for Teaching Theory

1. Choose teaching/learning theories that best fit a particular course or content and student learners.
2. Actively engage students in the content you're teaching as often as possible.
3. Include emphasis in all classes on the health professions' core competencies: patient-centered care, interdisciplinary teams, evidence-based practice, quality improvement, and informatics.

Questions for Further Reflection

1. How do theory, technology, and clinical teaching principles mesh to create quality health care in the future?
2. What are the implications of theory, technology, and best practices on your own self-directed, lifelong learning practices?

Learning Activity: Introductory Letter to Students

How does adult education theory (or another theory) help you think about your own approach to teaching and learning? Are the concepts similar or different to your plans for working with students in a technology-rich setting? Imagine that you have an opportunity to share your theory of education in the form of a letter to current (or future) students for a specific class you will teach. Write an introductory letter to students about your class, sharing your approaches to teaching and learning. Include comments about how technology will be used in your class. As you write your letter, what aspects of adult education (or other) theory guide you?

Online Resources for Further Learning

- University of Michigan, Center for Research on Learning and Teaching. This site contains an index of educational theories, as well as links to additional theory sites: http://www.crlt.umich.edu/tstrategies/tslt.php
- National League for Nursing. This site describes hallmarks of outstanding education, including categories such as students, faculty,

curriculum, and teaching/evaluation strategies: http://www.nln.org/excellence/hallmarks_indicators.htm

■ University of Colorado–Denver, School of Education. This site presents information on modern theorists, including a section on concept mapping under constructivism: http://carbon.ucdenver.edu/~mryder/itc_data/idmodels.html#constructivism

REFERENCES

Billings, D. M., & Connors, H. R. (2009). *National League of Nursing (NLN) living book: Best practices in online learning.* Retrieved October 16, 2009, from http://www.electronicvision.com/nln/chapter02/index.htm

Carnegie Mellon University. (2009a). *Enhancing education: Teaching principles.* Retrieved October 16, 2009, from http://www.cmu.edu/teaching/principles/teaching.html

Carnegie Mellon University. (2009b). *Enhancing education: Learning principles.* Retrieved October 16, 2009, from http://www.cmu.edu/teaching/principles/learning.html

Chickering, A. W., & Gamson, A. F. (1987). *Seven principles for good practice in undergraduate education.* Retrieved October 16, 2009, from http://honolulu.hawaii.edu/intranet/committees/FacDevCom/guidebk/teachtip/7princip.htm

Chinn, P. L., & Kramer, M. K. (2004). *Integrated knowledge development in nursing* (6th ed.). Hong Kong: Mosby.

Finkelman, A., & Kenner, C. (2009). *Teaching IOM: Implications of the Institute of Medicine Reports for nursing education* (2nd ed.). Silver Spring, MD: American Nurses Association.

Institute of Medicine. (2001). *Crossing the quality chasm.* Washington, DC: National Academies Press.

Institute of Medicine. (2003). *Health professions education: A bridge to quality.* Washington, DC: National Academies Press.

Kaufman, D. M. (2003). ABC's of learning and teaching in medicine: Applying educational theory in practice. *British Medical Journal, 326,* 213–216.

Knowles, M. (1980). *The modern practice of adult education. From pedagogy to andragogy* (2nd ed.). Englewood Cliffs, NJ: Prentice Hall.

Savery, J. R., & Duffy, T. M. (1995). Problem based learning: An instructional model and its constructivist framework. *Educational Technology, 35,* 31–38.

Zimmerman, B., Plsek, P., & Lindberg, C. (2008). *Edgeware: Insights from complexity science for health care leaders.* Irving, TX: Plexus Institute.

4 Technology Teaching and Lesson Planning

CHAPTER GOAL

Gain practical tips for translating course content into instructional form, using lesson plans to focus the use of technologies.

BEGINNING REFLECTION

1. How would you rate your experiences and comfort with writing lesson plans?
2. Are you comfortable in helping students prepare for class, leading them through class, and then challenging them to use the materials as they leave?
3. How will you consider using technologies to engage students in learning?

INTRODUCTION

This chapter is about organizing a plan to make technology an efficient part of our teaching and your students' learning outcomes. Why does a lesson plan help us make sense of our work in teaching with technologies? Technology won't solve all teaching problems, but, particularly with a new generation of student learners, it may provide useful tools for engaging students in learning. Lesson plans help us think about and choose reasonable options for using technology to accomplish learning purposes. Lesson plans provide a thoughtful approach to our teaching and can help us decide when and if technologies serve to enhance learning. Lesson plans make teaching more than a random act; they can make teaching a purposeful activity that can be evaluated and developed further over time.

LESSON PLANS AS ORGANIZING TOOLS

A lesson plan is considered a guide for teaching/learning plans. Lesson plans come in many shapes and sizes, but in almost all cases they influence our classroom accomplishments. Using the road map analogy, we need to map out where we are going with our teaching/learning plans, or there is a good chance we won't reach the destination efficiently and effectively. Lesson plans provide a way to capture and organize our content and our plans for helping students learn. Many components go into lesson planning, and these components provide ways to organize ideas into meaningful classes. Technologies provide opportunities to consider different approaches to teaching/learning. While lesson plans provide the written organized format for a class, technology often supplies the hands-on, active approach to teaching/learning. It is important to put technology into the lesson plan only when it provides the best learning experience. Lesson plans provide direction for a class and remind us why and how technology will be used to accomplish class objectives.

Lesson plans convey a way to organize our thinking, helping us choose from among a variety of options for teaching a concept. Technology can promote efficiency and effectiveness in considering and organizing materials. For example, how many ways can diabetic foot care be taught? What are the best approaches for a particular student group? The learning activity in this chapter outlines some ideas to think about with this process. As we begin the diabetic foot care exercise, it is essential to think about who our learners are, what their particular learning needs are related to learning diabetic foot care, how best to accomplish the teaching/learning activity, whether a selected technology will be useful, and what the anticipated outcomes should be.

THE INTEGRATED LEARNING TRIANGLE AS GUIDE

Lesson plans help organize our classes. The Integrated Learning Triangle provides direction, helping us make the best choices among the many ways that content can be taught. For example, if faculty are preparing to teach a class on wound care, there are many considerations regarding ways this can be taught and ways that technology can be included. Wound care lectures, videos, clinical labs, and review of Web sites or readings about wound care with electronic quizzes are examples of some of the many ways. All these uses clearly provide learning opportunities, but we as faculty, as well as students, all have finite amounts of time to accomplish our learning purposes. Choosing the best learning options for a given context is what lesson plans help us do. The Integrated Learning Triangle for Teaching With Technologies is one tool for further developing our technology-supported lesson plans. Concepts within the Integrated Learning Triangle diagram are further elaborated to guide lesson planning on a variety of topics.

It is particularly important to consider the context for learning. Because all nursing classes are different, the logistics, resources, and context remind us to focus on who our learners are, what resources are available for teaching/learning (including time frames and people resources), and needed learning outcomes. Context also reminds us to set a particular course within the context of a course curriculum (building on prior learning and creating a path to further learning in future classes).

Points of the triangle remind us to assess where learners are (related to the content), what their needed learning outcomes are, what teaching/learning activities might best help them achieve these outcomes, and what feedback is needed to keep learning on track. In the wound care example, very basic considerations include beginning students versus more advanced, simple versus complex wound care outcomes, and what type of learning activities might best fit this context.

A FORMAT FOR LESSON PLANS

Organizing the content for a lesson plan is sometimes challenging because of the myriad content that exists in nursing. Once topical areas are determined, concept mapping provides one tool to help organize lesson plans and classes (Walker Teaching Resource Center, 2002). These maps help us consider the important concepts to be taught and their relationships.

They serve as a useful tool in organizing the must-know content for students. In the text *Understanding by Design* (Wiggins & McTighe, 1998), the authors recommend a template approach to course and lesson planning that begins with the desired outcomes and works backward to objectives and learning activities. Others use an outline format as the easiest way to summarize a lesson plan. A one-page visual class organizer can serve as a lesson plan and a communication tool (Lenz, 1998). In rapidly changing clinical arenas, complexity theory suggests that broad questions can guide us in determining content to be considered (Zimmerman, Plsek, & Lindberg, 2008).

Diverse formats can be used for sharing lesson plans; there is no one right way. Thinking about the lesson plan as a communication tool (for yourself and others) provides direction in plan development. For example, you will want the lesson plan to be specific enough that others would know what should be covered, what strategies should be used to do the teaching, including use of technologies, and how learning outcomes should be evaluated. Often one specific, school-wide, lesson plan format is developed by a faculty team.

Once student learning needs are identified, a lesson plan can be built that includes the following commonly used categories:

- Outcome statements/objectives
- Organization of must-know content or key themes
- Active teaching/learning plans (including appropriate technologies) to engage learners
- Evaluation and feedback plans

Within the category of active learning, additional questions we will be incorporating into planning related to technologies include the following:

- Is technology required to accomplish the outcomes/objectives?
- Would technology enhance teaching/learning?

OUTCOME STATEMENTS AND OBJECTIVES AS LESSON PLAN ORGANIZERS

Within lesson plans, outcome statements/objectives serve as key tools. They provide a frame for the class and help faculty (as well as students) stay on track and accomplish what was intended. Just as there are many different types of picture frames to frame a picture (each varied picture frame showcasing the picture in a bit different way), there are many different ways to frame a lesson (and many different ways to incorporate technologies into the lesson plan picture).

Student outcomes are determined based on student characteristics and needs. These outcomes will vary based on the level of our students and the type of content we are trying to convey. Once determined, the outcomes provide the framework for creating appropriate teaching/learning strategies that are based on best teaching evidence. Outcome statements, broad statements of learning intention, provide direction in teaching/ learning. The example of a teenager learning to drive a car provides an example of three commonly accepted learning categories:

- Affective learning (appreciating ethical responsibilities with driving)
- Behavioral learning (demonstrating actual driving ability)
- Cognitive learning (knowing the rules of the road)

Bloom's (1956) taxonomy, a classic reference, is one guide to writing objectives and provides broad direction for leveling the cognitive outcomes/objectives to be asked of students. Web resources abound for assistance in creating class objectives. A quick Internet search for "Bloom's taxonomy" can help you identify guides to use in developing and evaluating

Exhibit 4.1

SELF-ASSESSMENT TO EVALUATE WRITTEN OBJECTIVES

When writing objectives, a few things to self-assess for include the following. Were you able to:

- Keep objectives specific enough to measure but broad enough to allow some flexibility in the class?
- Avoid overly relying on common verbs like *describe* and *identify?*
- Make your objectives as action-oriented as possible and as high a level in Bloom's taxonomy as appropriate for your learner?
- Include affective verbs like *value* and *appreciate?*
- Include objectives that allow students to complete the ABCs specific to the class topic: affective/valuing, behavioral/doing, and cognitive/knowing?

your objectives. Additionally, see Exhibit 4.1 for a self-assessment to evaluate written objectives.

CLARIFYING AND ORGANIZING THE MUST-KNOW CONTENT

How much content is too much? How much is enough? At a time of information overload, faculty can avoid trying to teach everything in the books by focusing on the must-know concepts for specified classes. A national dialogue on organization of learning materials via broad concepts supports helping students learn conceptually with exemplars versus trying to memorize long laundry lists of information. Again the advent of PDAs and quickly accessible information provides students fingertip access to detailed points of unusual disease symptoms or medication interactions.

The American Association of Higher Education document on ethical issues in education (Murray, Gillese, Lennon, Mercer, & Robinson, 1996) describes the faculty role in being content knowledgeable. The rapid advances in clinical knowledge challenge faculty to constantly stay updated on the breadth of subjects we teach. The advent of technologies supports work, by helping each faculty member be a seeker of information.

As noted, thinking about content and thinking about objectives go hand in hand. Adult education theory reminds us to focus on what the learners need to know, relevant to their current or future practice (Knowles, 1984). Guides for how to make presentations clear are summarized by McKeachie and Svinicki (2006) and include beginning with simple, familiar concepts, using multiple examples, and eliminating nonessential information. Sample ways to begin organization can be facilitated with technology such as using electronic concept maps and organizers. Additionally consider the following points:

- Emphasize key points (via broad concepts as possible).
- Keep material manageable and logically organized.
- Use the chunking approach to organize information.

If we start with the basics or the main concepts to be covered, helping the learner understand why these concepts are important, we can then build more specific information onto that base. For example, you might have a learning objective to help students understand the broad concept of anti-inflammatory drugs rather then having students try to outline and memorize specific drugs. Appropriate questions can help guide our thinking. For example, beginning questions specific to the learners' needs incorporate the affective, cognitive, and behavioral learning domains:

1. What values or attitudes are needed by students?
2. What specific factual information is needed?
3. What specific behaviors are needed?

For example, in a class about strategies to promote older adults' self-care for medication management, students need to appreciate the fact that promoting self-care is important, they need to learn simple strategies (such as cueing techniques) that can promote older adults' self-care, and they should be able to demonstrate these self-care promotion strategies in their work with patients.

ADDITIONAL CONSIDERATIONS: PRE-/POSTCLASS LEARNING AND TECHNOLOGIES

Pre- and postclass learning activities in our lesson plans support and encourage significant learning (Fink, 2003). The concept of creating both introductory set and closure helps capture these ideas within a lesson plan. Technology then provides opportunities for additional assignments, helping students capture further details or nice-to-know information beyond the classroom.

Creating Set for a Class Session or Presentation

Introductory set, just like it sounds, includes setting the stage for learning. Set includes helping students prepare for class, such as preclass assignments, and then setting a positive tone for learning once students arrive at class. Technology has enhanced our opportunities for supporting students' preparation for class. Students can electronically submit items such as learning quizzes, key points from readings, or brief paragraphs about their experiences with a topic before class begins. Once students arrive at class (whether classroom or online) the first few minutes of your class time (or introductory materials if online) set the stage for learning. Examples include synthesizing points from student preclass submissions, sharing a story about the topic to engage their interest, and highlighting the major points to be gained from the presentation. Clickers or automated response systems also support opportunities for learning quizzes in class based on assigned readings.

Creating Closure for a Class or Presentation

Closure, just like it sounds, involves getting the most from the closing minutes of your class (or closing communications if online); this step includes strategies such as summaries and review questions. This step provides the opportunity to reinforce content one last time. Fink (2003) additionally recommends using this time to challenge students in how they will use the information gained as well as helping students set further learning goals. In a classroom this step might include setting aside the last 10 minutes of class to use reinforcement strategies. In an online class this "what next?" step might be conveyed through a final summary of module activity. This can also remind students of further learning resources for opportunities to expand learning.

ACTIVE LEARNING AND TECHNOLOGY TO ENGAGE THE LEARNER

Once we have identified class objectives, there are numerous ways to achieve them. Our goal is to enhance our skills at providing content to students in ways that help students understand, remember, and apply the information. Complexity theory (Zimmerman, Plsek, & Lindberg, 2008) reminds us that there are numerous pathways and processes for students to gain successful learning outcomes.

Using a variety of interactive teaching strategies helps meet the needs of a diverse audience. Bean (1996) summarizes a variety of tools that serve as assignments in engaging students in active learning, including ideas for active writing assignments and problem-based learning. A combination of teaching strategies keeps presentations interesting and perhaps even fun. An interactive component to the educational program promotes students' participation in learning. Remembering basic educational principles helps determine which of the following combinations of learning approaches (many based on technologies) best fit your learners' needs.

- **Verbal or Audio Strategies.** Use lecture judiciously as an important tool for conveying selected facts. Incorporate questions for thought or discussion into lectures to promote interest and increase their effectiveness. For example, in a classroom lecture on self-care, describe briefly the specific communication techniques that can be used to promote self-care, and then build in questions that help students frame and solve problems using that information.

■ *Visual Strategies.* Provide multiple sensory cues about a topic, such as adding a visual component to the spoken word, to promote students' understanding and retention of information. Help students understand why the topic is important for the patients they care for by using imagery techniques. It is often helpful to build on basic strategies of watching a technique or process, whether by video or in real-time.

■ *Kinesthetic or Doing Strategies.* Individuals often learn best by doing; practice can make the link between the facts presented and the actual clinical application of those facts. Role playing or simulations can be a warm-up for the clinical practice experience or an alternate approach when actual supervised practice is not practical. Supervised practice in a learning lab setting or the clinical setting promotes the opportunity to check off learning competencies.

The preceding activities noted are the basis of many technologies. As we consider basic presentation plans, we think about our use of active

Exhibit 4.2

FIRED-UP TEACHING

Use the following concepts to light a FIRE for your class teaching:

Focused program content
■ Emphasize key points.
■ Make content relevant and easily applicable.

Interactive teaching strategies
■ Use a variety of strategies to meet the needs of diverse audiences.

Reinforced learning
■ Share information repeatedly from a variety of perspectives.

Evaluated learning
■ Help students identify what they have learned.

learning strategies that promote student engagement and critical thinking. A variety of interactive strategies, such as discussion questions, case study, and role play, can be used to promote practice and retention of materials. Another approach includes using the mnemonic FIRE to guide lesson planning (see Exhibit 4.2, "Fired-up Teaching"). The letters remind us to use *f*ocused program content, *i*nteractive teaching methods, *r*einforced learning, and *e*valuation. Using this tool, a variety of adult education principles for promoting teaching/learning are incorporated into a class session.

EVALUATION AND FEEDBACK

Assignment blueprints and evaluation templates are keys to a successful class. According to Walvoord, Anderson, and Angelo (1998), what students have to do to earn an A should be the same as what students have to do to learn well. This concept works in guiding both teaching practices and evaluation. In future chapters, evaluation concepts are discussed in more detail. Strategies for developing an assignment and evaluation blueprint based on lesson plan outcomes/objectives are then discussed. Concepts for evaluating lesson plans are provided in Exhibit 4.3.

Exhibit 4.3

LESSON PLAN SELF-ASSESSMENT CHECKLIST

A few self-assessment points to consider when developing lesson plans follow. Have you considered:

1. Assessing your learners' differing needs, learning styles, and knowledge backgrounds?
2. Stating specific objectives/expected outcomes (recalling that there are multiple ways to meet these)?
3. Organizing the must-know content in a reasonable outline format?
4. Enhancing motivations to learn by creating introductory set and learning incentives?
5. Asking learners to prepare and actively participate in your classes?
6. Using multiple approaches to enhance learning?
7. Incorporating evaluation into your lesson plan?

As discussed previously in the chapter, the evidence-based review abstract "Best Practice for Orienting Students to Learning" is provided in Exhibit 4.4. This synthesis of best evidence provides further direction for our work as educators.

Exhibit 4.4

EVIDENCE-BASED REVIEW ABSTRACT: BEST PRACTICE FOR ORIENTING STUDENTS TO LEARNING

Compiled by: Suzanne Stricklin, MSN, RN

The Challenge

Much of course and clinical orientation for undergraduate nursing students is rote in nature, with limited student appreciation. Several hours of class time and entire clinical days are spent on this topic, yet students do not feel as if their questions have been answered. Instead, many feel overwhelmed and believe the instructor is asking the impossible. Learning takes on new and exciting avenues every day, yet our orientations have not followed. Students are crying for assistance in how to sort through the extensive amount of information presented, but little time is dedicated to addressing such issues. The purpose of this abstract is to establish a framework for student orientation that allows for maintaining high expectations and excellence, while giving students what they need to be successful.

Synthesis/Interpretation of Literature

While a systematic literature review revealed that limited literature exists on this topic, findings included: (a) exercises geared toward specific course objectives are helpful when new areas are being introduced, (b) specific high-risk groups may need additional orientation geared to their particular needs, (c) anxiety may be a useful topic (especially test anxiety) to address (though research is not con-clusive), (d) students want communication with peers and faculty that is not just cursory, (e) leave out most of the administrative information (provide this another way), (f) use of mastery-oriented teaching practices when introducing material promotes increased persistence, (g) when faculty are introduced, encouragement of help-seeking is essential and it needs to be followed up regularly thereafter, (h) introduction of specific study strategies may increase success, (i) weeklong orientations may promote success in some populations, (j) presenting the same material in each class may lead to student boredom and limited retention, and (k) Students want substantive content early.

Brief Model Case

Application of this evidence could be accomplished by providing new faculty with an opportunity to assess their current personal knowledge, followed by exploring

(Continued)

Exhibit 4.4

EVIDENCE-BASED REVIEW ABSTRACT: BEST PRACTICE FOR ORIENTING STUDENTS TO LEARNING (*Continued*)

best practices in orienting students. They could be asked to gather previously used orientation plans/materials or develop a list of items they believe should be included in the orientation of a course they are teaching in the upcoming semester, including who, what, when, where, how, and why. Following presentation of the evidence, faculty could be asked to rethink their orientation plans and to identify specific changes they will make, based on the evidence.

Bibliography

Arnault-Pelletier, V., Brown, S., Desjarlais, J., & McBeth, B. (2006). Circle of strength. *Canadian Nurse, 102*(4), 22–26.

Dearing, K. S., & Steadman, S. (2008). Challenging stereotyping and bias: A voice simulation study. *Journal of Nursing Education, 47*(2), 59–65.

Edelman, M. (2005). A measure of success: Nursing students and test anxiety. *Journal of Nurses in Staff Development, 21*(2), 55–61.

Gardner, E. A. (2006). Instruction in mastery goal orientation: Developing problem solving and persistence for clinical settings. *Journal of Nursing Education, 45*(9), 343–347.

Goldworthy, S. J., Goodman, B., & Muirhead, B. (2005). Goal orientation and its relationship to academic success in a laptop-based BScN program. *International Journal of Nursing Education Scholarship, 2*(1). Retrieved October 16, 2009, from http://www.bepress.com/ijnes/vol2/iss1/art22/

Lee, C. J. (2005). Academic help seeking: Theory and strategies for nursing faculty. *Journal of Nursing Education, 46*(10), 468–475.

Stevenson, J. M., Buchanan, D. A., & Sharpe, A. (2006/2007). Commentary: The pivotal role of the faculty in propelling student persistence and progress toward degree completion. *Journal of College Student Retention, 8*(2), 141–148.

Thompson, M. K., & Consi, T. R. (2007). Engineering outreach through college pre-orientation programs: MIT discover engineering. *Journal of STEM Education, 8*(3&4), 75–82.

Tynjala, P., Salminen, R. T., Sutela, T., Nuutinen, A., & Pitkanen, S. (2005). Factors related to study success in engineering education. *European Journal of Engineering Education, 30*(2), 221.

Weeks, L., Calderon, E., Chappell, J. A., & Caver, P. E. (1986). A hospital experiment in teamwork among students, nurses, and administrators. *Journal of Medical Education, 61*, 736–742.

Wilson, S. (2005/2006). Improving retention and success: A case study approach for practical results. *Journal of College Student Retention, 7*(3–4), 245–261.

Worrell, M. M. (2005). Packing a bag for the journey ahead: Preparing nursing students for success. *Inquiry, 10*(1), 49–50.

SUMMARY

Using lesson plans to organize classes can remind us to make technology an efficient part of our teaching and our students' learning outcomes. The lesson plan structure provides direction and guidance in preparing effective classes. Lesson plans incorporate outcomes/objectives, must-know content, and active learning assignments with appropriate technologies to engage learners and support learning evaluation.

ENDING REFLECTION

1. What is the most important thing you gained from this chapter?
2. What are your plans for using the information in this chapter in your future teaching endeavors?
3. What are your further learning goals?

GUIDELINES FOR TECHNOLOGY TEACHING AND LESSON PLANNING

Quick Tips for Lesson Plans

1. Package the lesson in a way other faculty can use or learn from (or that it can serve as a guide from semester to semester).
2. Integrate a variety of assignment types to meet diverse learner needs.
3. Gain input and critique from colleagues.
4. Use the Integrated Learning Triangle to help organize a class session or module.

Questions for Further Reflection

1. What is the role of lesson plans in preparing health profession students of the future?
2. In what ways can technology be used to promote ease of developing and sharing lesson plans?

Learning Activity: How Many Different Ways Are There to Teach Diabetic Foot Care?

How might you develop a lesson plan on teaching diabetic foot care? Consider the following questions as you think about the components to your plan:

- Should all classes on diabetic foot care be taught the same way?
- Is technology required to teach this topic?
- Could selected technologies enhance learning?
- Are students best taught by watching a video? By listening to a podcast? By demonstration and practice?
- Will you incorporate strategies that encourage critical thinking about diabetic foot care?
- Will you incorporate strategies that document diabetic foot care learning?

How many possible ways can you identify? Will you use a combination of approaches? How does the Integrated Learning Triangle (Appendix B) guide you in making these decisions?

Online Resources for Further Learning

- *Ten Ways to Make Your Teaching More Effective.* This resource provides ideas for ways to make an interactive presentation effective: http://teaching.berkeley.edu/tenways.html
- University of Kansas Center for Teaching Excellence. A variety of resources relevant to lesson planning for the beginning educator are provided: http://www.cte.ku.edu/index.shtml
- University of Victoria. *Bloom's Taxonomy, University of Victoria.* A synthesis of learning skills specific to varied levels of the taxonomy is provided: http://www.coun.uvic.ca/learn/program/hndouts/bloom.html

REFERENCES

Bean, J. C. (1996). *Engaging ideas: The professor's guide to integrating writing, critical thinking, and active learning in the classroom.* San Francisco: Jossey-Bass.

Bloom, B. S. (1956). *Taxonomy of educational objectives, handbook I: The cognitive domain.* New York: David McKay.

Fink, L. D. (2003). *Creating significant learning experiences: An integrated approach to designing college courses.* San Francisco: Jossey-Bass

Knowles, M. (1984). *The adult learner: A neglected species.* Houston, TX: Gulf Publishing.

Lenz, K. (1998). *The course organizer routine.* Lawrence, KS: Edge Enterprises.

McKeachie, W., & Svinicki, M. (2006). How to make lectures more effective. In W. McKeachie & M. Svinicki (Eds.), *McKeachie's teaching tips: Strategies, research, and theory for college and university teachers* (12th ed., pp. 57–73). Boston, MA: Houghton Mifflin.

Murray, H., Gillese, E., Lennon, M., Mercer, P., & Robinson, M. (1996). *American Association of Higher Education bulletin.* Retrieved October 16, 2009, from http://www.aahea.org/bulletins/articles/Ethical+Principles.htm

Walker Teaching Resource Center. (2002). *Concept mapping and curriculum design.* University of Tennessee, Chattanooga. Retrieved October 16, 2009, from http://www.utc.edu/Administration/WalkerTeachingResourceCenter/FacultyDevelopment/ConceptMapping/

Walvoord, B., Anderson, V., & Angelo, T. (1998). *Effective grading: A tool for learning and assessment.* San Francisco: Jossey-Bass.

Wiggins, G., & McTighe, J. (1998). *Understanding by design.* Alexandria, VA: Association for Supervision & Curriculum Development.

Zimmerman, B., Plsek, P., & Lindberg, C. (2008). *Edgeware: Insights from complexity science for health care leaders.* Bordentown, NJ: Plexus Institute.

5 Computer and Information Literacy: Gaining and Using the Evidence With Technology

CHAPTER GOAL

Consider information literacy as a critical concept in evidence-based practice (EBP) and identify tools/techniques to help students gain information literacy competencies.

BEGINNING REFLECTION

1. What does the concept of information literacy mean to you?
2. If you are currently teaching, how do you help your students search the literature? If you are not teaching, what is your approach to searching the literature?
3. How can your approach be updated to keep up with new access to information and technologies?

INTRODUCTION

Clinical education is rapidly changing, and our students and graduates need tools to keep up. The Web changes the amount of information we have to access as well as how we access that information. In the past, students likely prepared to care for patients by having one good textbook and hoping it covered the complexity of their patients. Now students can prepare, in essence, with a universe of knowledge that is open to them. The challenge is that they can become lost in that universe without some guidance. Now the textbook (digital or hardcopy) more likely serves as a basic guide, with additional Web sites required for further topic detail or ongoing updates.

Clinicians have been noted to have deficiencies in how to search, evaluate, and apply the best evidence (Institute of Medicine [IOM], 2003). Information literacy and EBP are two key concepts that can help bridge an education and practice gap. Varied nursing organizations recognize these as essential. For example:

- The *Essentials of Baccalaureate Education for Professional Nursing Practice* identifies computer skills and information literacy as competencies required by undergraduate nursing programs (American Association of Colleges of Nursing, 2008).
- The American Nurses Association (2008) has described information literacy as a critical concept in supporting EBP.

Information literacy concepts are also consistent with lifelong learning, which will be essential to all health care professionals and educators. The purpose of this chapter is to discuss information literacy as a central concept in teaching with technologies. The chapter describes steps to help both faculty and students use technology as a process for accessing information resources. Strategies for helping students access, critique, and use resources in meaningful ways are chapter themes.

INFORMATION LITERACY: WHAT DOES IT MEAN?

Information literacy serves as a tool and foundation for lifelong learning and a basis for further work with technologies. Information literacy has been described as a broad concept involving cognitive skills, application of technical skills, and knowledge (International Information and Communication Technologies [ICT], 2002). A description of information literacy based on work of the American Library Association (2009) includes the following:

- Knowing when information is needed
- Identifying the type of information needed to address a problem
- Finding and evaluating the information
- Organizing and using the information to address the problem

Concepts added to that include the following:

- Synthesizing accumulated information into an existing body of knowledge
- Communicating search results effectively and clearly
- Considering social issues and ethical aspects related to information dissemination (Jacobs, Rosenfeld, & Haber, 2003)

Why do some students find searching the literature confusing? Rapid advances in technologies such as the Web have led to almost unlimited access to information. While it is fairly easy to access vast amounts of information, it is more challenging to ensure that students understand the worth of that information and interpret it correctly. Data suggest that students experience the following challenges with information literacy (Appel, 2006):

- Identifying trustworthy and useful information
- Managing excessive information
- Effectively communicating information

With volumes of information available, the concepts and processes for attaining information literacy will be valuable for students' work in the future. Faculty have an opportunity to provide direction in learning this important skill.

RELATED CONCEPTS

Information literacy and EBP are overlapping concepts. Accessing and using literature efficiently relates to an evidence base for clinical practice. In terms of helping students work with patients, information literacy is consistent with EBP. Additional related terms include *reading literacy* and *health literacy*. These are similar-sounding but different concepts. All these terms are important in helping students and their future patients understand health information. Computer literacy is considered a component of information literacy. Descriptors of selected terms for discussion purposes include the following:

- *Information literacy* relates to skills or competencies needed to efficiently maneuver through the vast amounts of information available.
- *EBP*, in simple terms, means basing clinical practice on the best evidence available. The goal is to use evidence from a well-developed body of research. When research is missing, best evidence has been

extended to include best practices coming from theory and expert clinicians.

- *Research utilization* might be considered an extension of EBP to include a focus on using well-developed research as a basis for clinical decisions.
- *Computer literacy* involves managing the computer for skills required in information literacy.
- *Reading literacy* relates to general reading ability.
- *Health literacy* is the ability to read and understand with a specific focus on health-related issues (IOM, 2004).

HOW DO WE HELP STUDENTS LEARN INFORMATION LITERACY?

Update search methods to reflect available technologies. The concept of searching the literature has changed with the advent of the Web. When it comes to technology and information literacy, we ask students and future practitioners to take on new roles. We used to spend hours in the library with some version of a large cumulative index, then seek a copy machine for copies, and then make bibliography cards from those copies. With the wealth of information now online, that system has limited use. Students will be better served if we update the methods for teaching literature searching to reflect the new realities of technologies.

Help students understand why they must do literature reviews. A major focus involves helping beginning students understand why they are being asked to review the literature. Beginning students have often become accustomed to faculty or the textbook synthesizing the information they need to know. With literature searches, we ask students to transition from readers of texts to those who find and critique diverse resources. Fewer skills are needed to review a text that has all the information synthesized in one place than to create and critique a concept search from a variety of professional publications or Web-based resources (ICT, 2002).

Teach basic strategies for beginners and more advanced strategies for advanced students. The novice-to-expert model (Benner, 2001) supports transitions in gaining skills for information literacy and EBP. Competencies specific to an evidence-based skill set have been developed through the Academic Center for Evidence-Based Practice (Stevens, 2005). These competencies relate to a skill set for EBP with competencies designed specifically for varied program levels from undergraduate to doctoral.

Recognizing Professional Literature

Faculty may need to teach beginners how to recognize professional literature. Both faculty and students may wonder what counts as professional literature. There is an amazing variety of data sources available online, and the boundaries between professional and other types of data are often blurred. Further issues arise because print sources can often be accessed online. It is important that teachers help students to recognize what is and is not professional literature. For beginning students, this may be as basic as creating criteria by assignment type or stipulating that professional references should include an identifiable author, publication source, and date of publication.

Being Systematic in Finding and Accessing Information

Because so much data is accessible, as a part of information literacy faculty need to help students understand how to begin and refine literature searches. Technology makes it easy to access resources for guiding clinical practice, but finding the best resources can be challenging. Faculty can help students understand the basics of systematic review as a key component of information literacy. Use of electronic resources leads to the potential for promoting more efficient use of best evidence.

The mass of information available makes it impossible to review all of the literature. Instead, we should strive for a systematic review. Because technology has enhanced our access to the literature throughout the world, it is no longer possible to say we have consistently reviewed all of the literature. In the past it was common to note a thorough literature review was completed. Today's worldwide library makes it less clear what a thorough search entails. It is no wonder the changing concept of *search* may be confusing for students.

Systematic search means describing or making reproducible the search strategy (Fink, 2004). Faculty can guide students, particularly more advanced students, in the following ways:

- Describe what is meant by the term *systematic search* and why it is important.
- Frame the search. Framing includes describing concepts and terms used in the search as well as the databases searched. This also includes clarifying terms—that is, taking terms from a fuzzy concept to something recognizable in the literature.

- Be thoughtful about databases. Most students currently have access to a variety of databases and search options. Which databases are best for answering questions? The answer depends on the questions asked. Guide students in searching outside common professional databases as necessitated by the problem identified.
- Participate in discussions as to what counts as an acceptable literature/evidence source. This includes if and how diverse Web sites or other resources such as blogs or wikis fit. For example, will an assignment be directed toward students gaining professional references from traditional literature or will other resources be accepted?
- Partner with faculty/librarians for searches. Faculty/librarian teams are beneficial for developing assignments, framing searches, and tracking elusive publications.

Again, basic approaches are considered for beginning students and more advanced approaches for advanced students. This chapter's "Learning Activity" provides prompts about systematic review in a quiz type format that can be used as a beginning self-assessment of knowledge about systematic review. It can serve as a class discussion guide as well.

Thinking Critically and Critiquing

Confirm that students understand the different levels of evidence. Our teaching process varies with our student levels (considering their sophistication with research critique). A basic consideration for all students includes the ability to describe the level of evidence presented in a particular resource. This is as basic as confirming student understanding of the levels or types of information. For example, all students should understand that quantitative studies are at the highest end of a continuum and are followed by qualitative studies, institutional databases, and clinical expertise (IOM, 2003). The process for teaching further critique varies depending on student levels and the level of evidence available on topics of interest. The learning needs of the students guide the level of critique presented (again, basic students need basic approaches).

Synthesizing and Communicating

Synthesizing means combining the information found and making sense of the literature recommendations. It requires reflection and critical thinking and includes looking for strengths, weaknesses, or gaps in the litera-

Exhibit 5.1

FINDING THE EVIDENCE, SELECTED EVIDENCE-BASED PRACTICE, AND RESEARCH UTILIZATION GROUPS

Examples of formal evidence-based practice and research utilization resource groups can be found at the following:

■ The Cochrane Collaboration, Cochrane Reviews: http://www.cochrane.org/reviews/
■ Evidence-Based Practice, Agency for Health Care Policy and Research: http://www.ahrq.gov/clinic/epcix.htm
■ U.S. Preventive Services Task Force, Agency for Health Care Policy and Research: http://www.ahrq.gov/CLINIC/uspstfix.htm
■ Put Prevention Into Practice, Agency for Health Care Policy and Research: http://www.ahrq.gov/Clinic/ppipix.htm

---

ture evidence. This critical reflection guides students in making summary statements about the level of evidence from the various sources. A variety of resources exist for teaching critique strategies and helping students access best evidence online. Sample tools are included in Exhibit 5.1, "Finding the Evidence, Selected Evidence-Based Practice, and Research Utilization Groups."

CRITIQUE OF WEB-BASED RESOURCES AND OTHER MEDIA

There are many resources available to students online and many of these have been developed without professional peer review. Our discussion has focused primarily on professional print publications for critique, but, particularly as students seek online resources to review, options among these resources can become quite complex. We need to guide students in first differentiating between a range of online resources, varying from professional journal databases and Web sites to very basic lay information (with many shades between). Second, we need to assist students with guidelines for critical evaluation of these diverse Web resources.

Some of the various kinds of materials online are reliable and valid and some not. Beginning resources exist to help students learn to critique these diverse resources. While professional references such as journal

Exhibit 5.2

REVIEW CRITERIA FOR HEALTH INFORMATION ONLINE

The following provide guides to help students (and their patients) critique online resources related to health care:

- *A User's Guide to Finding and Evaluating Health Information on the Web Medical Library Association:* http://www.mlanet.org/resources/userguide.html
- *Evaluating Internet Health Information: A Tutorial from the National Library of Medicine:* http://www.nlm.nih.gov/medlineplus/webeval/webeval.html
- *Assessing the Quality of Internet Health Information,* Agency for Healthcare Research and Quality (AHRQ): http://www.ahrq.gov/data/infoqual.htm

---

articles and research on the Web use the noted criteria for literature critique, additional questions will relate to the reliability and validity of other types of resources such as lay and professional Web sites that students access. Students have extensive access to information that is quite unique, and it may help or hinder their professional efforts. Exhibit 5.2 provides resources to assist students with their review of health information online.

This same review process applies to the myriad online resources that exist in other formats (e.g., videos and podcasts) and with various uses (e.g., patient education resources, drug guides). Expanded guidelines for critiquing online videos are now emerging (MD Advice, n.d.). Stress to students the importance of determining whether these resources are quality products or simply commercials. Students will need to gain critique strategies for the varied resources now available online. Our approaches to information search and critique are obviously changing.

INFORMATION LITERACY AND EVIDENCE-BASED PRACTICE

How does EBP relate to information literacy and clinical practice applications? The goal of EBP is to gain and use best evidence in helping patients and providers make choices in clinical care to promote safety, quality, and health care value (IOM, 2003). In teaching students information literacy and EBP, we:

- Assess their current expertise or educational level,
- Orient them to both what they will be doing and why it is important,

- Engage them with relevant assignments that challenge (but do not overwhelm), and
- Provide feedback based on the student level.

Faculty can direct students to utilize evidence-based resources in developing their assignments, even with something as basic as guidance in developing a health fair poster. For example, as students seek references to support their poster, faculty help them identify the differences between a self-help page on the Web developed by one individual and the EBP resources from the National Institutes of Health or other national organizations. In asking students to use the best science (or evidence) in their projects, faculty might, for example, direct beginning students developing a depression awareness poster to use an appropriate evidence base such as the National Institutes for Health or the Centers for Disease Control.

As students advance with more complex assignments directed toward gaining an evidence base, critical thinking is enhanced as they consider the relevance of information they have searched and retrieved or syntheses they have found on a given topic. As search strategies were discussed earlier in this chapter, the focus now becomes the clinical problem and the population and context.

As we teach with technology we are trying to help students develop self-directed learning habits for lifelong learning. This is particularly important as related to gaining tools for information literacy and EBP. Students, for example, will find available online pamphlets they can provide to patients, but these will need to be based on the best evidence to be credible. A faculty role includes helping students use best evidence in clinical decision making for needed practice changes. Initially faculty can help students to:

- Understand the need to identify and frame the clinical problem. This can be as basic as how to frame a clinical question to obtain the best literature search or evidence base. The mnemonic PICO (Patient, Intervention, Comparison, Outcome) can be taught, for example, to help frame clinical questions (Melnyk & Fineout-Overholt, 2005).
- Begin clinical topic searches seeking systematic reviews, recalling the benefits of well-done systematic review on a given topic.
- Think critically and consider the relevance of information students have searched and gained or syntheses they have found on a given topic.
- Evaluate evidence-based protocols for appropriateness for specific specialty populations.

The same evidence-based protocol may not be useful in all settings nor for all patients. While information literacy is about locating and evaluating information, EBP supports clinical decisions in the context in which they are applied. After gaining the best evidence on a topic, students also need to learn to put the evidence gained into context, applying information appropriately to a given patient population and setting. Fall prevention is one example. While basic fall prevention concepts are relevant across settings, specific fall prevention protocols depend not only on physical environments but on patient characteristics. For example, for a patient with Parkinson's disease, the protocols would differ depending on the stage of the disease and the patient setting (e.g., home or hospital). Exhibit 5.1, discussed earlier in the chapter, provides further resources.

THE WEB, PERSONAL DIGITAL ASSISTANTS, AND OTHER FINGERTIP TECHNOLOGIES

Fingertip technology is a term used to describe easy access to our clinical information. Mobile computing devices such as personal digital assistants (PDAs), smartphones, and notebook computers can be used in systematic search and retrieval of evidence-based protocols at points of care. Strategies for gaining the evidence via these technologies are the same as described earlier, including search strategies and evidence critique. The main advantages to fingertip technologies are portability and clinical point-of-care access. Particularly for students who are still learning the basics, these tools provide an important way to rapidly access information for changing patient needs. Many interest groups, including hospitals, specialty groups, and governmental agencies, are intent on exploring how technologies can promote information literacy and a strong evidence base to enhance patient care quality. These devices can also assist clinicians in providing quality care through point-of-care clinical documentation.

CREATING ALLIANCES

Creating partnerships or alliances with librarians and other health professionals is a suggested approach to combining and enhancing knowledge and expertise. Mutually beneficial opportunities for creating educational projects are described (Jacobs et al., 2003). Benefits to these partnerships include the following:

- Communicating and collaborating. Teaming up with librarians reminds us what services are available and provides a good start to systematic reviews. The American Library Association (2009) provides numerous resources of benefit in guiding student learning.
- Reviewing evidence developed by other disciplines. We have opportunities for multiple disciplines to share and learn from each others' professional literature, helping students best understand the state of the science on a topic area. Real benefit exists in adding a frame or perspective of another discipline in viewing and enhancing our evidence base for practice. See Exhibit 5.3, "Sample Health Professions Databases and Electronic Resources."

The concept of learning how to find and use resources for answering questions or solving problems has been addressed by MacKay, Millis, and Brent (2006). They provide recommendations such as the following:

- Partner with librarians in developing orientation sessions or modules.
- Work collaboratively in developing clear project assignment guidelines.
- Include pathfinders to help students get started in literature searches.

Exhibit 5.3

SAMPLE HEALTH PROFESSIONS DATABASES AND ELECTRONIC RESOURCES

CINAHL

What It Is: broad selection of nursing and allied health citations
Key Features: links to full-text if available, e-mail alerts available

Access Medicine

What It Is: online collection of medical reference books and tools
Key Features: includes drug guides, images, patient care, decision-making tools, and patient education

Cochrane Library

What It Is: a collection of databases designed to provide evidence for decision making
Key Features: excellent resource for systematic reviews

(Continued)

Exhibit 5.3

SAMPLE HEALTH PROFESSIONS DATABASES AND ELECTRONIC RESOURCES (*Continued*)

ProQuest Nursing & Allied Health Source

What It Is: database of nursing and allied health citations
Key Features: includes Joanna Briggs Institute evidence-based best practice information sheets, systematic reviews, and evidence summaries

PubMed

What It Is: searchable medical literature database covering selected international biomedical journals
Information Provided: clinical and biomedical literature citations
Key Features: links to online full-text, clinical queries, and e-mail alerts are available

MedlinePlus

What It Is: searchable full-text consumer-level health information database
Key Features: encyclopedia, dictionaries, images, clinical trial information, and tutorials

TRIP: Turning Research Into Practice

What It Is: searches numerous evidence-based resources
Key Features: offers evidence-based medicine, images, and patient information searches

Adapted with permission from Whitehair (2009).

- Include the use of student critique partners to critique appropriateness of resources.
- Sequence project assignment parts with intermittent deadlines for providing students' feedback.
- Include assessment tools such as rubrics and make use of peer review.

SUMMARY

As clinicians emerge from our educational programs, it is important that they have skills for information literacy and know the process for EBP to serve as good clinicians for their patients. In the health professions education report (IOM, 2003), a quality gap is described as the care patients receive versus the care patients should receive. Information literacy and EBP, based on informed clinicians knowing how to access the best practice knowledge, is one contribution to narrowing that quality gap. Once we as faculty have helped students understand the basics, such as what counts as professional literature, our focus will be to help them think critically about both the process for searching and the criteria for critique. Faculty provide guides that help students understand what professional literature is, find the best clinical evidence, critique it, and apply the information in appropriate contexts.

ENDING REFLECTION

1. What is the most important content that you learned in this chapter?
2. What are your plans for using the information in this chapter in your future teaching endeavors?
3. What are your further learning goals?

GUIDELINES FOR COMPUTER AND INFORMATION LITERACY: GAINING AND USING THE EVIDENCE WITH TECHNOLOGY

Quick Tips for Evidence-Based Practice

1. Involve librarian partners in working with students to enhance their search skills and broaden their information literacy.
2. Create assignments that help students identify the ways that an evidence base is currently used in their clinical setting (e.g., reviewing protocols or clinical pathways on a topic).

Questions for Further Reflection

1. Where does information literacy belong in the curriculum?
2. What are the similarities and differences in learning needs related to EBP for beginning health professions students and advanced graduate students?
3. How do we integrate the concept of EBP across a curriculum so that all faculty are moving in the same direction? Are there best practices to guide us in this endeavor?

Learning Activity: Systematic Review and Seeking the Best Evidence Survey

Answer "agree" or "disagree" to each of the following statements related to literature review seeking best evidence on a topic.[1]

1. ____A practical screen and methodological screen for including/excluding articles in literature reviews are the same thing.
2. ____An online literature search is typically a sufficient approach to the review of the literature.
3. ____Searching one database should cover most educational research topics.
4. ____Finding the key words in an article title makes this a good match for your literature review.
5. ____Descriptive reviews rely on reviewer experiences and evidence, while a meta-analysis uses statistical techniques to combine study results.
6. ____A decision trail relates primarily to your research methods section.
7. ____A literature review is systematic, explicit, and reproducible.
8. ____Inclusion and exclusion criteria are important concepts for a literature review.
9. ____A screening protocol can promote consistency and quality in a review.
10. ____Descriptive reviews identify and interpret similarities and differences in literature purpose, methods, and findings.
11. ____A standardized review protocol can be helpful in clarifying inclusion/exclusion criteria.
12. ____When completing a literature review, once your search criteria are set, no changes should be made.
13. ____Once a research literature review is completed, a synthesis report should be generated to summarize and identify themes and gaps in the literature.
14. ____In completing literature reviews, it can be useful to develop a matrix that allows one to organize results by topics such as type of article and year of publication.

---

[1]Survey concepts developed from Garrard (2006). Responses 1, 2, 3, 4, 6, and 12 are considered "Disagree"; all others are considered "Agree."

15. ____After completing a descriptive literature review to answer specific questions, the reviewer has a responsibility to disseminate and make the information as accessible as possible.

Online Resources for Further Learning

- American Library Association. This association provides a variety of resources on information literacy and tips for working with students: http://www.ala.org/
- Academic Center for Evidence-Based Practice (ACE). This center provides diverse online resources for educators as well as ongoing workshops on teaching EBP: http://www.acestar.uthscsa.edu/

REFERENCES

American Association of Colleges of Nursing. (2008). *The essentials of baccalaureate education for professional nursing practice.* Retrieved August 31, 2009, from http://www.aacn.nche.edu/Education/bacessn.htm

American Library Association. (2009). *Information literacy competency standards for higher education.* Retrieved October 12, 2009, from http://www.ala.org/ala/mgrps/divs/acrl/standards/informationliteracycompetency.cfm

American Nurses Association. (2008). *Nursing informatics: Practice scope and standards of practice.* Silver Springs, MD: Author.

Appel, J. (2006). Students struggle with information literacy. *eSchool News.* Retrieved August 31, 2009, from http://www.eschoolnews.com/resources/measuring-21st-century-skills/measuring-21st-century-skills-articles/index.cfm?rc=1&i=42042

Benner P. (2001). *From novice to expert, commemorative edition.* Upper Saddle River, NJ: Prentice Hall Health.

Fink, A. (2004). *Conducting research literature reviews: From paper to the Internet.* Beverly Hills, CA: Sage Publications.

Garrard, J. (2006). *Health sciences literature review made easy: The matrix method* (2nd ed.). Boston, MA: Jones & Bartlett.

Institute of Medicine (IOM). (2003). *Health professions education: A bridge to quality.* Retrieved October 10, 2009, from http://www.nap.edu/catalog.php?record_id=10681

Institute of Medicine (IOM). (2004). *Health literacy: A prescription to end confusion.* Retrieved October 10, 2009, from http://www.iom.edu/?id=19750

International Information and Communication Technologies (ICT) Literacy Panel. (2002). *Digital transformation, a framework for ITC literacy.* Retrieved August 31, 2009, from http://www.ets.org/Media/Tests/Information_and_Communication_Technology_Literacy/ictreport.pdf

Jacobs, S., Rosenfeld, P., & Haber, J, (2003). Information literacy as the foundation for evidence-based practice in graduate nursing education: A curriculum-integrated approach. *Journal of Professional Nursing, 19*(5), 320–328.

MacKay, G., Millis, B., & Brent, R. (2006). *IDEA objective 9: Learning how to find and use resources for answering questions or solving problems.* Retrieved August 31, 2009, from http://www.theideacenter.org/sites/default/files/Objective9.pdf

MD Advice. (n.d.). *Video medical news.* Retrieved October 10, 2009, from www.mdadvice.com/news/video.html

Melnyk, B. M., & Fineout-Overholt, E. (2005). *Evidence-based practice in nursing and healthcare: A guide to best practice.* Philadelphia, PA: Lippincott Williams & Wilkins.

Stevens, K. (2005). *Essential competencies for evidence-based practice in nursing.* San Antonio, TX: Academic Center for Evidence-Based Practice, the University of Texas Health Science Center.

Whitehair, C. (2009). *Sample health professions databases and electronic resources.* Unpublished manuscript, University of Kansas Medical Center.

Faculty as Learning Facilitators With Technology

6   Technologies and Effective Communication

CHAPTER GOAL

Consider good communication practices to guide teaching with technologies and facilitate communication in a variety of situations.

BEGINNING REFLECTION

1. How does technology affect your current communications?
2. What are your current communication approaches when teaching with technologies for different purposes and for different audiences, such as individuals versus groups?

INTRODUCTION

Communication is the cornerstone of our relationships with others. Be it verbal, nonverbal, handwritten, text-based, in person, or virtual, communication provides the means by which people convey their thoughts, feelings, and ideas to others. Communication ranges from the most personal and intimate communication to the most impersonal and indifferent.

In today's world it often feels that there is no escape from the constant barrage of incoming messages. Technology makes it possible to reach anyone, anyplace, anytime. There are more and more communication options available to us, from cell phones and text messages to communication within learning management systems. How do we keep up with all the possible means of communication? How do we manage the influx of messages and respond appropriately in content, manner, and time? Given the 24/7 nature of today's communication, how do we somehow manage the sheer number of messages needing a response? Which ones take priority?

On a very different but equally important note, how can technology be used to communicate effectively with our students and health care communities? With the muting of facial expressions, gestures, and vocal inflections across video or computer screens, or their absence in the case of text-based communication, the effectiveness of communication can be limited. This stripping away of nonverbal communication can leave meaning more difficult to interpret. Communication is oftentimes complicated further by differing opinions, values, perspectives, cultures, and languages. Add to this complexity the potential life-and-death nature of health care–related conversations, and the importance of good communication for nurses becomes apparent.

WHY IS COMMUNICATION IMPORTANT IN TEACHING TECHNOLOGIES?

Communication is important as the cornerstone of relationships with students and peers, as a tool to facilitate learning and critical-thinking skills, and as a mechanism by which to improve the safety and quality of patient care. Communication "focuses on how people use messages to generate meaning within and across all kinds of contexts, cultures, channels and media" (National Communication Association, 2009). Communication is a learned process that consists of verbal, nonverbal, and electronic messages. Health care communication is often complicated by the life-and-death, hierarchical, and legal aspects of health care itself. Today those complexities have increased with the explosion of technologies that offer to facilitate, but can just as easily derail, communication efforts. Faculty are called upon to be good communicators in a variety of situations, with a variety of individuals or groups, using a variety of technologies.

Relationships

Effective communication is an essential element in the teacher–student relationship. Faculty must be able to communicate clear expectations to individual students as well as to groups of students. Of course, students have a responsibility to express any confusion and ask questions when faculty expectations and direction are not clear, but, again, the faculty must then respond with clear direction. The onus is on faculty to communicate clearly, concisely, and appropriately, all in a timely manner.

It is also up to faculty to model professional communication to their students. Role modeling professional communication includes a broad range of skills, including collegial communication with peers, interdisciplinary communication within health care teams, and direct communication with patients. Among its five core competencies, the Institute of Medicine (IOM, 2003) recommends that the education of health care professionals include interdisciplinary teamwork, in which members learn to work together to achieve patient outcomes. It also recommends education in the use of informatics to facilitate communication, reduce errors, and improve patient outcomes.

Learning and Critical Thinking

Communication has traditionally been used to evaluate how much learning has taken place. Students have been asked to communicate, via paper and pencil tests, online multiple choice exams, and formal papers, the extent to which they have mastered required content. What is often less recognized is the importance of communication to the learning process itself. For example, writing activities can be used not only to evaluate learning but also to facilitate the learning process. Online, text-based discussions are examples of written assignments that can be used to teach critical-thinking skills.

Safe, Quality Patient Care

Good communication skills are essential to safe, quality patient care. Perhaps this truth is best recognized in its absence. "Communication failure, a leading source of adverse events in health care, was involved in approximately 75% of more than 7,000 root cause analysis reports to the Department of Veterans Affairs National Center for Patient Safety" (Dunn et al.,

Exhibit 6.1

HEALTH LITERACY RESOURCES FOR FURTHER LEARNING

- *Health Literacy.* Resources are provided by the Health Resources and Services Administration, including free programs for online training: http://www.hrsa.gov/healthliteracy/
- *Health Literacy, a Prescription to End Confusion.* An online text from the Institute of Medicine provides a variety of readings to guide students in learning to improve their work in health literacy: http://www.nap.edu/catalog.php?record_id=10883

2007, p. 317). This statistic highlights the fact that teaching students improved communication skills is essential and can directly improve the quality of health care.

Health Literacy

The concept of health literacy is central to safe patient care, especially when communicating and teaching with diverse patients. Concepts of health care literacy are central to patient education, with cultural diversity, health literacy, and patient teaching being intertwined topics. As noted, communication failures are considered to be a major problem in current health care systems. Teaching health literacy skills is particularly important because once students have gained comfort with health care vocabulary they may not remember that these terms are often confusing to patients. Students will have limited impact on patients, health care systems, and public health without a focus on health literacy. Sample resources for helping students gain skills in health literacy are provided in Exhibit 6.1.

TEXT-BASED, COMPUTER-MEDIATED COMMUNICATION

Computer-mediated communication has become such a major factor in our world that entire journals such as the *Journal of Computer-Mediated Communication* are devoted to this topic. As often happens as technology evolves, semantics can be problematic because the technology changes so rapidly. While many text-based communications are computer mediated, that is not always true (i.e., this book is text based but not computer mediated). Conversely, many computer-mediated communications are text based but, again, that is not always true (i.e., podcasts and Skype). Our focus here is on communication that is both text based and computer mediated.

Text-based, computer-mediated communication can be either synchronous or asynchronous. *Synchronous* means that the people in communication with one another are communicating at the same time, while *asynchronous* means that the parties are not required to communicate with one another at the same time. These terms have been used extensively in online education but can have relevance in other venues as well. Public and private communications are additional categories to consider. We can focus on communication to an individual or convey messages to groups, large or small. Eduscapes (2008a) provides further comments specific to online communication.

As text-based, computer-mediated communication replaces communication that was previously verbal, the expectations and uses of writing itself are changing. It used to be that most verbal communication was casual, and written communication was often more formal. Now, although formal writing (such as scholarly papers) still exists, much written communication is more informal, and the standards for traditional, formal writing do not fit this new informal written communication style. For example, proper nouns and names are frequently not capitalized, and slang acronyms (such as "LOL," for "laughing out loud") abound. The transition from traditional, formal writing styles to contemporary, more informal writing styles presents a challenge for faculty, as students come with a focus on text-based lingo and faculty try to determine what is acceptable professionally.

Fortunately there are a growing number of practice guides for the differing technological options available. A good, broadly based communication guide that applies across all situations including the Internet is found in Shea's (1994) book, *Netiquette,* in which she identifies 10 core rules that still serve well in most cases. These rules, like theoretical foundations and best practices, remain fairly constant regardless of the specific text-based communication used. For example, Shea reminds us that, even in cyberspace, there is a human being at the other end of our communication, and that person deserves to have their time and privacy respected. Equally important is to use the same standards of behavior online that you would use in person. These are fundamental concepts, to be sure, but they are still relevant with today's technology.

GUIDES FOR COMMUNICATING WITH STUDENTS

While the explosion of technology provides an opportunity to use any of a large variety of technological options for any given communication, the general principles of good communication apply regardless of the form of communication used (even old fashioned, face-to-face communication). New technologies do mean, however, that faculty are in the position of having many choices, and they need to make informed, responsible decisions. Sometimes the simplest of those decisions are the hardest. For example, how does one handle the multiple messages (be they phone or text-based messages) that arrive daily from students? Basic tips include the following:

1. Make informed and responsible decisions on the mechanism by which you respond to students. Just because a student e-mailed you does not mean you need to respond via e-mail. Sometimes a quick phone call is the best way to clarify complicated questions or situations.
2. Clarify to whom you should respond. If you are responding to a student with information that everyone in a course needs to know, then use a communication technique capable of including the entire class in the response. If you are responding to a student with personal or negative information, respond only to the individual directly.
3. Respond at a set time each day, limit that time, and tell students what your communication schedule is. One strategy used to manage the constant barrage of e-mails is to ignore the temptation to read and respond to them all day long. If you answer e-mail once a day at noon, tell students so that they know what to expect; if you plan to avoid or limit weekend responses, let students know that is your practice.
4. Give extra thought to the delivery of bad news (such as negative feedback on a paper or a poor grade). Blunt comments via text-based communication can come across as scathing, so take precautions to soften the message or use a face-to-face (or some other

form of verbal communication) method that provides more input than simply the words used.

5. Pick the mode of your communication to fit the situation. Verbal communication provides noted benefits, but if you want a written record of sending the message and its receipt, e-mail can be a good option. Conversely, if you do not need a paper trail of the communication, or risk its being sent to someone else, then do not write it down.

ADDITIONAL CONSIDERATIONS WITH COMMUNICATION

Writing Assignments

Writing is one of the best critical thinking activities and hence the concept of writing to learn has become commonplace. Traditionally we have thought of writing as a mechanism to demonstrate and evaluate the completion of the learning process, such as end-of-semester term papers. These final products are considered high-stakes writing, because they are usually graded only one time for accuracy, completeness, and scholarly format. An example is the term paper that is due toward the end of a course and that often represents a large portion of the course grade. An alternate approach is to require the same term paper assignment but design it to be completed in parts throughout the semester. Breaking the paper down into smaller assignments provides an opportunity for students to gain feedback along the way and learn by making improvements to the assignment prior to submitting the entire paper at the semester's end. This step-by-step approach would be considered a lower-stakes form of writing evaluation.

But *writing to learn* also refers to the use of writing as a key component of the learning process. Here the purpose is not to document completed learning but to facilitate the learning process itself, such as through journaling. In this case, the purpose of the writing is to stimulate thoughts and connections between content and to engage students with the content to be learned. Such writing is usually informal, messy, and not edited to perfection. It is not graded per se, though credit may be given for its completion. This low-stakes writing offers many benefits, such as identifying misunderstandings, improving discussion, providing practice in writing, providing individualized insight into each student, and improving more formal writing projects.

Class Discussions

Basic principles of discussions hold true regardless of the technological format used or even if the discussions are face-to-face in classrooms. Discussions across settings are prone to the same issues, such as how prepared students are (or are not) for the discussion and how much the instructor should (or should not) participate. Although discussions have long been used as learning tools, online discussions have forced faculty to become more conscious and explicit in communicating guidelines to students. Some tips to direct discussions (whether classroom or online) include the following:

1. Determine the purpose of the discussion and how best it should be orchestrated. Using objectives, such as with a lesson plan format, provides direction for gaining desired outcomes.
2. Orient students to course discussion guidelines, including the expected frequency of student participation and the extent of participation recommended.
3. Clearly define your role as faculty in the discussion and communicate that to students. Too much faculty participation can smother a discussion, but too little can result in misinformation or wandering off topic. Particularly in online discussions, let students know when they can expect to hear from faculty.
4. If the class is large, breaking up into smaller groups can be helpful. Optimal group size can vary depending on the nature of the discussion, but group size should be compatible with the discussion purpose and type and the amount of participation recommended.
5. Provide clear and concise evaluation criteria so that, if students are to be graded on a discussion, they know the criteria. Faculty decisions about criteria include all aspects of participation that will be evaluated, such as how often to respond and the quality of response. A simple rubric can outline faculty expectations.
6. Use interesting prompts and pose focused, open-ended questions to begin discussions and keep the discussions going. Sample prompts are provided by Eduscapes (2008b).

FEEDBACK AND EVALUATION

Keeping a focus on the desired learning outcome for the students, which is the overall goal of the communication, promotes feedback as a learning tool. Providing questions and prompts to promote communication with the student can facilitate the ongoing learning process.

Discussed in more detail in Chapter 9, feedback and evaluation are related (and sometimes overlapping) yet different processes. *Feedback* is the more general term in which comments and data about an action, behavior, or knowledge are designed to positively affect that action, behavior, or knowledge in the future. Feedback has been described as information communicated to students that is based on an assessment and that helps students reflect and work further with the information provided. This includes constructing self-knowledge relevant to course learning and setting further learning goals (Bonnel, Ludwig, & Smith, 2007). Evaluation is the systematic appraisal (of value, rightness, accuracy, appropriateness) of an action, behavior, or knowledge.

Shea's (1994) rules of netiquette remind us that, although many of today's communication techniques use impersonal gadgets, there is a person on the other end of our communications and we need to treat him or her with the requisite respect all humans deserve. The opportunity to soften bad news, through face-to-face or video mechanisms that afford more than just textual input, is important to keep in mind. At the very least, reading and rereading and editing the text-based message before sending it helps assure that the message is softened as much as possible.

SOCIAL LEARNING SPACES AND SPECIAL COMMUNICATION SITUATIONS

New communication opportunities can also lead to new challenges. Many faculty and students belong to social spaces such as Facebook. The increased interest in social networking may actually blur professional and personal boundaries. The question becomes whether it is appropriate for faculty to have access to students' personal profiles and, conversely, if students should have access to faculty members' personal profiles. The open, public nature of these sites and the enduring nature of written words could create potential problems if communication does not meet high professional standards.

Consistent with the Ethical Principles for College and University Teaching (Murray, Gillese, Lennon, Mercer, & Robinson, 1996), guidelines of appropriate boundaries between students and faculty need to be followed. Attention needs to be paid to how or if a particular social space is relevant to educational uses. Faculty and students may have differing opinions on how to best use this type of technology in learning. If faculty decide to share pages with students, thoughtful consideration as to what personal content is posted is recommended. A related issue is faculty access to students' sites. Situations have been reported where students have posted inappropriate information (for example, exam questions and confidential information about patients) on their profiles. Such behavior becomes open to disciplinary action against these students. Whatever approach is taken, at the very least, the use of online social sites must be addressed in student orientations and through ongoing reminders.

Perhaps a broader view is needed. Skiba (2006) notes that, in the past, *learning spaces* referred primarily to classrooms. However, in today's virtual world, learning spaces are understood to be any place where learning occurs. In this respect, social spaces offer one more opportunity for a learning space, and the challenge for educators is to make the best possible use of that space for the most appropriate learning experiences and content. Further work by Skiba, Connors, and Jeffries (2009) suggests the benefit of social networking tools created by faculty to support ongoing communities of practice, including students as well as professionals. Ideas for using virtual spaces to support learning communities are further discussed in Chapter 7, "Technology Teaching Strategies and Building the Learning Community."

Faculty also need to remain cognizant of students with special needs. One such group might be students for whom English is a second language (ESL). Many ESL learners benefit from the nonverbal cues that visual communication and body language provide. Text-based communication, stripped of nonverbal cues to augment the words, is often more difficult for ELL students to interpret. Online technologies however do provide the opportunity to review archived discussions and to look up words in dictionaries. Evolving translator resources and online voice application technologies provide further opportunities for ESL students.

Technology-facilitated communication can be helpful to some students with special needs. The hearing impaired may benefit from text-based communication. Online courses may be particularly convenient for students with mobility impairments. Even students with impaired digits, hands, or limbs may benefit from voice-activated technology that enables them to participate more fully in courses. Further study of best approaches is needed.

HEALTH CARE IMPLICATIONS

Good communication techniques are key not only in the classroom, but also for preparing students to work on clinical teams. Communication has a tremendous impact on the quality of health care. The IOM reports (Finkelman & Kenner, 2009) have focused on quality care issues, paying particular attention to fragmented care and problems of communication within health care teams and between health care providers and patients that have had a negative impact on quality health care. "If there were one aspect of health care delivery an organization could work on that would have the greatest impact on patient safety, it would be improving the effectiveness of communication on all levels—written, oral, electronic" (HealthCare Benchmarks and Quality Improvement, 2002). For example, handoffs (when a patient's care is transferred from one health care provider to another) are recognized as high-risk periods often accompanied by inadequate communication (HealthCare Benchmarks and Quality Improvement, 2005). Technology systems have been touted as a major approach to reduce communication errors. For example, computerized medical records and prescriber order entry systems can promote safety by eliminating messy handwriting.

Computer-generated reminders can help reduce errors of omission. Online databases improve quality by ensuring that health care providers have access to the latest in evidence-based practice, and computerized decision support systems can help standardize approaches. Electronic medical records can make data more complete by highlighting missing data and can make that information available instantaneously to other members of the health care team and to the patient. Communication itself can be facilitated by using e-mail. Our students are prepared for clinical patient care only if they have comfort and skills with clinical technologies that enhance team communication.

SUMMARY

The imperative for students to learn clear communication skills in their courses is apparent. The need for good communication tools is broad and applies not only in education but also in leading discussions, clinical conferences, and in team meetings for patient care. We want to make communication as efficient and effective as possible. Communication tools will continue to evolve, and tools of lifelong learning will be needed to help gain strategies that best benefit our work with students. Good communication techniques are key both in our classrooms and for preparing our students to work on clinical teams.

ENDING REFLECTION

1. What is the most important content that you learned in this chapter?
2. What are your plans for using the information in this chapter in your future teaching endeavors?
3. What are your further learning goals?

GUIDELINES FOR TECHNOLOGIES AND EFFECTIVE COMMUNICATION

Quick Tips for Teaching

1. Remember the importance of introductions at the beginning of all classes to begin building the learning community (no matter what the technology focus of the course is).
2. Take the time early on to set the tone for frequent and friendly communications throughout the course. Use pictures of members of the learning community in courses where students are not seen to serve as a reminder of the human component.
3. Provide communication guides at the beginning of a course, telling students what to expect in respect to communication from you: for example, that you will respond to e-mail within 24 hours, or dates that you'll be out of the office with limited e-mail access.
4. When writing a difficult e-mail to a student, have a trusted colleague read it for feedback and also reread it a bit later yourself (or, preferably, both) before sending it.

Questions for Further Reflection

1. What ways can technology be used to help promote clear, consistent communication between students and faculty?

2. What ways can technology be used to help promote clear communication for patient care safety in the clinical setting?

Learning Activity

Writing activities are versatile and lend themselves to a variety of feedback options, all of which encourage the development of critical thinking skills in students. Looking at the list of writing-to-learn activities below, add as many new ideas as you can (challenge yourself to add three at first, and then increase that by increments of three each time you succeed):

1. Write a focused summary of the day's reading assignment.
2. Identify a problem statement for the day's topic.
3. Write a letter to another student about the topic.
4. Write a project notebook.
5. Write a journal over time about the topic.
6. Write either a response paper or a synthesis paper.
7. End the session with a 5-minute writing exercise about what was learned that day (the main idea).

Online Resources for Further Learning

■ University of Virginia, Teaching Resource Center. This site provides links to numerous teaching tips that transcend the technology used, including writing: http://trc.virginia.edu/Publications/Teaching_Concerns/TC_Topic/Writing.htm
■ University of California, Santa Cruz. Not focused specifically on teaching with technology, this site contains principles for good student discussions that cross technologies: http://ctl.ucsc.edu/resources/tips/index.html
■ National Communication Association. This site has several sections of relevance to teaching and learning, including "Education" and "Research" sections: http://www.natcom.org/

REFERENCES

Bonnel, W., Ludwig, C., & Smith, J. (2007). Providing feedback in online courses: What do students want? How do we do that? *Annual Review of Nursing Education, 6,* 205–221.
Dunn, E. J., Mills, P. D., Neily, J., Crittenden, M. D., Carmack, A. L., & Bagian, J. P. (2007). Medical team training: Applying crew resource management in the Veterans

Health Administration. *Joint Commission Journal of Quality Patient Safety*, 33(6), 317–325.

Eduscapes. (2008a). *Teaching and learning at a distance, course communication*. Retrieved May 30, 2009, from http://eduscapes.com/distance/course_communication/index.htm

Eduscapes. (2008b). *Teaching and learning at a distance, course discussion: Prompts*. Retrieved May 30, 2009, from http://eduscapes.com/distance/course_discussion/prompts.htm

Finkelman, A., & Kenner, C. (2009). *Teaching IOM: Implications of the Institute of Medicine Reports for nursing education* (2nd ed.). Silver Spring, MD: American Nurses Association.

HealthCare Benchmarks and Quality Improvement. (2002). *Poor communication is common cause of errors; communication critical, says JCAHO official—Joint Commission on Accreditation of Healthcare Organizations—brief article*. Retrieved September 29, 2009, from http://findarticles.com/p/articles/mi_m0NUZ/is_2_1/ai_90683346/

Healthcare Benchmarks and Quality Improvement. (2005). *JCAHO to look closely at patient handoffs: communication lapses will be key focus*. Retrieved September 29, 2009, from http://findarticles.com/p/articles/mi_m0NUZ/is_12_12/ai_n15998737/?tag=rbxcra.2.a.44

Institute of Medicine. (2003). *Health professions education: A bridge to quality*. Washington, DC: National Academies Press.

Murray, H., Gillese, E., Lennon, M., Mercer, P., & Robinson, M. (1996). *American Association of Higher Education bulletin*. Retrieved January 15, 2009, from http://www.aahea.org/bulletins/articles/Ethical+Principles.htm

National Communication Association. (2009). *Communication defined*. Retrieved October 10, 2009, from http://www.natcom.org/index.asp?bid=1339

Shea, V. (1994). *Netiquette*. San Francisco: Albion Books.

Skiba, D. J. (2006). Think spots: Where are your learning spaces? *Nursing Education Perspectives*. Retrieved October 8, 2009, from http://findarticles.com/p/articles/mi_hb3317/is_2_27/ai_n29262131/?tag=content

Skiba, D., Connors, H., & Jeffries, P. (2009). Information technologies and the transformation of nursing education, *Nursing Outlook*, 56(5), 225–230.

7

Technology Teaching Strategies and Building the Learning Community

CHAPTER GOAL

Gain tools for helping the learning community as a group to accomplish common learning goals.

BEGINNING REFLECTION

1. What is your definition of a learning community?
2. What are your best experiences participating in a learning community?
3. What goals do you have for facilitating learning communities?

INTRODUCTION

Learning is often considered a social activity. The need for contribution and relationships in learning as well as the important aspect of social and emotional learning are well noted (Carnegie Mellon University, 2009).

In learning communities, course members bring diverse perspectives for learning together and can enhance learning for all. Learning communities provide opportunities for collaborative problem solving, a sense of connection, and acknowledgment for contributions (Brookfield & Preskill, 2005). While learning communities are not a new phenomenon, the popularity of online education has led to increased attention to this concept. This chapter describes tools faculty can use to help diverse student communities learn with technology support.

In this text, learning communities are considered to be groups of people engaged in common learning goals. Dufour and Eaker (1998) described a professional learning community as including an environment that supports mutual cooperation, personal growth, emotional support, and synergy of efforts. Palloff and Pratt (2004) note that the concept of a learning community relates to more than knowledge gain or sharing; rather, the concept relates to an entire culture of learning. They describe a web of learning that includes not only concepts of content and technology but also student, peer, and faculty learning participation.

While the concept of learning community is often used to describe online learning, the concept has relevance across a broad range of teaching settings. Learning communities also help to promote the social aspect of face-to-face learning. As students share with each other as members of learning communities, they contribute to and strengthen collegial learning, providing a different approach to gaining knowledge (Vella, 2002). Additionally, being part of a learning community includes professional responsibility and being a good course citizen. Technology is a tool for engaging student learning communities and promoting learning.

Some learning community connections and activities are stronger than others. Learning community activities vary from individuals coming together to create new projects that meet learning objectives or to learn by sharing diverse experiences. While any classroom might be considered a learning community, those classrooms with strong student interaction geared toward mutual learning goals most closely fit the descriptor. From a constructivist perspective, students within learning communities share their learning experience, and others benefit as well. While many different purposes are noted in the following examples, all might be groups coming together for learning purposes, and any of the following might represent a learning community.

- Associate degree nursing students working in small groups to develop posters for their community college health fair

- A graduate student group that meets face-to-face for two days and then participates in an online listserv to share challenges and successes as they develop their skills on a clinical topical area
- Students working on a quality assurance project in a long-term care practicum to focus on preventing spread of infection

Several concepts are somewhat related to but different from the concept of the learning community as addressed in this text. The concept of a learning organization, for example, relates specifically to learning that is organization based and consists of paid employees working in groups on specific organizational problems. The concept of learning community has also been used to describe students who live together in a university setting to foster learning goals. The concept of online social communities is also popular, but these entities relate more to interactions and social networking than to learning tasks. These concepts and descriptors are not included in this discussion.

Learning communities can energize learning, moving learning from an isolated pursuit to a shared experience that helps students integrate concepts and make learning connections. Students learn to think about concepts differently as others share their experiences and examples. The example of differing approaches of two unique online geriatric courses conveys the concept of a learning community. In the first course, students write weekly papers, submit them to faculty for feedback, and receive a grade, all with total lack of knowledge of other students in the course. In a second course, students learn about each others' geriatric interests and goals for the course via introductory activities, a variety of assignments such as group activities, shared experiences, and topical discussions as the course progresses. While approaches for each course might be justified, enormous learning opportunities are missed in the first course by not bringing the community together for learning.

Diverse student groups, learning purposes, and settings make each learning community unique. Settings for learning communities can vary from online classes to face-to-face classrooms, learning labs, and clinical settings. Learning communities can be directed toward learning content varying from obstetrics to long-term care of the older adult. While this chapter focuses on the learning community in educational settings, faculty want to prepare students for broad clinical learning communities that work together to solve clinical practice problems as well. Working as part of clinical teams is one of the health professions educator report recommendations (Institute of Medicine [IOM], 2003). Technologies such as those supporting online discussions provide unique opportunities for diverse health professions students to meet for interdisciplinary conversations. A goal in health professions education is to move education and practice closer together since we are preparing students to work together in health care organizations.

As students work together in learning communities, relationships between learners can be strengthened via community approaches to gaining knowledge. Students gain focused opportunities to interact and participate in peer activities, learning together and providing feedback to each other. Feedback from faculty as well serves in connecting learning community activities with furthering learning goals. Questions and challenges generate continued learning.

Faculty can provide direction in helping the learning community work together. Acknowledging diverse learners, considering their roles as community members, providing good direction, and facilitating students' work are important concepts. Principles of good group work based on systems theory (Sampson & Marthas, 1990) provide the background for further discussion.

DIVERSE LEARNERS IN THE LEARNING COMMUNITY

Part of being a good teacher is knowing you have something new to learn about students at any given point in time and place (Bain, 2004). We find diversity in the classroom, in clinical settings, and in online courses. It is important to consider diverse students' needs not only to support learning together but also to help them prepare for their future work as diverse clinicians working together in clinical settings. Group and team learning will be an ongoing need in clinical settings (IOM, 2003).

Viewing our classes from the perspective of diverse students, we consider that diverse students are good for the course. We also seek to create a course that is good for diverse students. Human interactions make up all parts of our lives. Because learners are holistic beings, the social and emotional aspects of the classroom affect their learning (Carnegie Mellon University, 2009). Special attention is paid to group interactions. Concepts of collaboration and groups are key in course work that is centered around learning communities, allowing opportunities to learn from diverse learners.

One reason to consider student diversity in learning with technology is that a given technology may be less familiar to some populations because of cultural, age, and generational differences. Having a basic understanding of our students' backgrounds, interests, and educational attainment provides important context as we seek to move the learning community forward. Understanding the population provides direction in coaching and in providing optimal student learning resources.

Multigenerational Diversity

When we consider diversity, we need to consider how different generations come together and learn. Diverse generations of learners bring unique ways of being in the world. They bring different perspectives on what is important, how to learn, and how to work together. Diverse generations have learned in different ways with different tools. Groups who often need to learn and work together include the Millennials (those born in 1980s to early 1990s); Generation Xers (those born from the mid 1960s to late 1970s); and the aging Baby Boomers (Oblinger, 2003). For example, opportunities for students to participate in, interact with, experience, and construct knowledge to meet their own learning needs are consistent with learning styles of the new Millennial student generation but often vary from styles of other cohorts (Skiba, 2005). The unique needs and perspectives of each of these groups are worthy of attention when planning to teach with technologies.

Technologies and Diversity

We also see diversity in students' technology skills and enthusiasm for technology. Diverse generations have been described in various ways, including the net generation or digital natives, those who have grown up using technology, as distinguished from the non-net generation or digital immigrants, those who gain technology skills later in life (Skiba, 2005). The digital divide also describes the differences between those individuals who have access to technology and those who do not (Young, 2001).

While access to technologies in the home setting has improved, faculty have a responsibility to provide alternate access methods if technology ownership is not a requirement of a program. Typically we are seeing more comfort with technologies, but technologies can still be challenging for some learners, in particular the digital immigrants who find technologies a new way of doing things.

Cultural Diversity

Students making up our learning communities are becoming increasingly diverse, including not only diverse ethnic backgrounds but also diverse socioeconomic backgrounds. These unique mixes of students can vary from those who are heads of households to those who are parent supported. Online education in particular has few geographic boundaries and has made programs more accessible, promoting opportunities for a larger pool of students to participate together. Diverse students bring unique background experiences and provide different perspectives on the larger world. Benefits include learning from a variety of perspectives as students young and old learn from each others' experiences and stories.

To work effectively with diverse students, understanding the importance of broad definitions of diversity to fit our changing classrooms is an important starting point. Being mindful of the uniqueness of each student, being open-minded, and using diverse teaching strategies are good beginnings to try to meet a variety of learning needs. Ethical teaching principles described by the American Association of Higher Education (Murray, Gillese, Lennon, Mercer, & Robinson, 1996) stress the importance of being sensitive to diverse student needs and preparing for and debriefing potentially difficult learning situations. Resources for helping faculty consider diversity are available, providing further ideas for thoughtful approaches to teaching and learning. (See Exhibit 7.1, "Resources for Working With Diverse Students.")

Exhibit 7.1

RESOURCES FOR WORKING WITH DIVERSE STUDENTS

- "Diversity and Complexity in the Classroom." This chapter from the Barbara Gross Davis book, *Tools for Teaching*, provides a variety of practical strategies to work with a variety of diverse students, many of which can be applied to teaching and learning with technologies: http://teaching.berkeley.edu/bgd/diversity.html
- *Enhancing Diversity in the Nursing Workforce.* This resource summarizes current challenges in creating a diverse workforce and suggests strategies to enhance diversity in both the classroom and the workplace: http://www.aacn.nche.edu/Media/FactSheets/diversity.htm

BUILDING OUR LEARNING COMMUNITIES

Learning communities often complete work in groups. Nursing education and group assignments create an interesting mix. Putting students in groups does not automatically create collaboration. Group work has been described by numerous students as challenging. Examples of the challenges faced by groups of students, as reported in the literature, include unclear assignments, unwieldy group size, and social loafing (Kroen & Bonnel, 2007). Faculty members report their own challenges in facilitating online groups and grading group projects, such as clarifying group member project contributions.

Faculty take on roles as group facilitators in supporting the learning community. Group theory (Sampson & Marthas, 1990) provides a broader background for working with learning communities, building on systems theory and including concepts such as group development, group norms, and group structure and roles. Beginning considerations for successful groups, such as orientation, readiness for group activity, and peer evaluation, are provided in the literature (University of Sydney, n.d.). Fink (2003) notes that well-developed assignments and prompt feedback do much more to help teams improve their functioning than does teaching them about group interaction. Further tips for using groups effectively, such as promoting individual accountability and stimulating idea exchange within groups (Michaelsen, 1998), are provided in diverse online resources.

Since different needs are apparent at different points in the semester, suggestions for each phase are outlined in the following sections. A focus on group beginnings, middles, and ends provides beginning direction in organizing work with our learning communities.

Beginnings

Course beginnings provide the opportunity to bring groups together with common interests and to help prepare students to be successful. Each unique student cohort brings fresh perspectives to learning at a given point in time. Technologies provide opportunities to help group members get to know each other. Introductory activities provide faculty as well as students with opportunities to learn about others and gain confidence in sharing. Diverse needs, abilities, and learning styles of each unique group can be ascertained to provide direction for guiding students in accomplishing learning goals. Suggested activities include the following.

Group Introductions and Surveys of the Class

Whether prior to class or at the beginning of a classroom session, technologies provide opportunities to gain a quick snapshot of the students in the course as well as to create opportunities for group connections. Group introductions and introductory surveys can highlight a group's characteristics, including basic demographic data such as age, background, and interests. Additionally, reflective preclass questions can be generated that vary by topic studied. For example, asking students a very basic question about their experiences working with patients with Alzheimer's disease prior to a class on dementia serves as a type of assessment.

Depending on the setting, students can use e-mail, course management systems, or classroom clickers to complete these simple introductions and surveys. As students reflect and share, they begin to take more responsibility for learning and faculty gain a better understanding of students' background and learning goals.

Orienting and Setting the Stage for the Learning Community

The beginning class session or module can be used to orient students to the workings and the value of being part of a learning community as well as creating set for the class. A good student orientation includes an introduction to the learning community concept and the work of the class—not just the class content but the activities as well (Palloff & Pratt, 2004). Conveying the information that all students will be working together and gaining from each others' experiences and perspectives provides beginning direction. Orientation can do the following:

- Convey benefits of active participation in learning
- Share guidelines for student responsibilities to participate in discussion and share with colleagues
- Provide tips for giving peer feedback (peer activities are particularly important ways to help students gain needed peer-review skills for the future)

Middles and Transitions

The goal of learning communities is to work together in learning, so assignments need to be designed to promote this outcome. As students are transitioning through often large amounts of information and projects, the possibility of losing momentum exists. The faculty facilitator role provides opportunities to help the class maintain momentum. Being proactive in assignment/course design and using good facilitator skills to engage with and encourage students promotes successful transitions throughout the assigned project or course.

Providing Assignments That Allow Mutual Learning Opportunities and Sharing

Being proactive with good class design that engages learners promotes easier transitions and fewer challenges throughout a class session. Building in varied interaction modes helps meet diverse learner needs. If group projects are part of the class, guides include helping groups be clear on objectives, how students will divide tasks, and what the final product will be. Peer review can be a component. Sharing interviews or observations, working on team projects via portfolios, and discussions are useful tools in promoting group learning. Asking students to share experiences and perspectives promotes reflection, further learning, and relationships between learners; this also helps students gain perspectives on others' views of the world.

Using Social Spaces

Online social spaces may provide opportunities for student assignments and networking as the course progresses. Depending on institutional guidelines, resources such as LinkedIn and Twitter may provide ways for students to reflect on their experiences and share with others. Further Web resources for considering these options are provided in this chapter's "Online Resources for Further Learning" section.

Serving as Facilitator for the Learning Community

Facilitating learning builds on good assignments and course design within a course that is focused on a student learning community. Facilitation includes faculty roles in engaging and encouraging students for ongoing learning within the community and assisting the community in accomplishing learning objectives. Students learn that faculty are present as course facilitators who promote group interactivity through the various group phases (Palloff & Pratt, 2004).

Synthesizing and Summarizing

Faculty summarize and keep the community moving forward via feedback on discussions and shared activities. This ongoing/periodic feedback to the learning community acknowledges emerging learning and connects activities with the goal of furthering learning. This includes reminding students of accomplishments to date and providing further questions and challenges that still need to be addressed.

Endings

Endings include reflection and debriefing as a group. These activities help students prepare for closure and further goal setting, whether at the conclusion of an assignment or the end of the semester.

Build in Reflective Opportunities

Sharing reflections about what has been learned via active class participation helps promote student learning. Wiggins and McTighe (1998) noted that an isolated learning activity does not lead to understanding but that reflection on the activity itself helps promote understanding.

Provide Synthesis of Learning Accomplishments

Faculty can synthesize class accomplishments and relate these to overall class learning goals. This summary leads naturally to the "What next?" questions and can help students prepare for closure and further goal setting. For example, in an online class, a simple content analysis completed by faculty and an e-mail summary of key themes from Web discussions provide the benefit of debriefing and providing feedback to students. Themes noted from discussions help summarize work and create links to past and future course content. Faculty serve as course guides in providing these summaries that also allow highlighting of discussion points, help students make conceptual connections from student examples, and bring closure to a topic.

BEING A GOOD COURSE CITIZEN: THE ETIQUETTE OF LEARNING TOGETHER WITH TECHNOLOGIES

In today's technology-rich classroom, both face-to-face and online, civility and digital citizenship are important community concepts. Students take on community membership to some degree in all courses, regardless of the course type. Students learn that being good community members includes acknowledging professional roles and rules for good citizenship with technologies. While relevant across all technologies, this topic is particularly important in online classrooms, as there may be added challenges if face-to-face communication benefits are missing. The International Society for Technology in Education (2004) standards include three broad topics related to learning together with technologies:

- Developing positive attitudes toward technology applications that support collaboration, lifelong learning and productivity
- Understanding the ethical, cultural, and societal issues related to technologies
- Practicing responsible use of technology systems, information, and software

While varied technologies present different citizenship issues, concepts of safety and security in the digital world are broadly applicable. Professional behaviors including respectful awareness of all learning community members are key. Faculty can be proactive with guidelines that promote good course citizenship and appropriate use of technologies for learning (rather than spending class time focused on problem solving). Besides providing students with an orientation to expected classroom roles, citizenship guides describing good citizenship standards can be provided. Ideas for developing guidelines for "digital citizenship" can be gained from a review of sample documents on the Web. Depending on the level of the class, concepts may be as basic as being respectful of each other and being responsible in the use of technology. Asking students to complete a digital citizenship audit that includes self-assessments of personal technology behaviors has been recommended (Ribble, Bailey, & Ross, 2004). General guidelines (Ribble et al., 2004) include the following:

- Take a prospective approach to developing a positive learning community.
- Orient students to school handbooks of professional conduct.
- Consider developing class civility documents.
- Ask students to sign technology codes of conduct that include broad guides for appropriate use of digital devices.

As health professionals, we have professional ethical guidelines to meet as well. In nursing, for example, the American Nurses Association provides ethical guidelines that direct ethical behavior in the profession. Consequences to all professions can be major if we do not address important ethical issues. With rapidly changing technologies in the classroom, all the rules for good citizenship have not yet been developed. Ribble et al. (2004) suggest continued questioning of what is and is not an appropriate use of technology, anticipating that our descriptions of what is appropriate will change over time.

SUMMARY

Learning communities have goals of learning together. Teaching goals include providing diverse teaching and learning methods for diverse learners as well as promoting professional, civic-minded learning communities. Attending to selected strategies with beginnings, transitions, and endings of course learning communities provides direction. As we prepare students for future clinical work, group learning situations provide practice for working in clinical teams. The varied settings in which our student learning communities will be expected to function provide impetus for our work. Learning communities can be powerful tools and take learning far beyond traditional classroom approaches.

ENDING REFLECTION

1. What is the most important content that you learned in this chapter?
2. What are your plans for using the information in this chapter in your future teaching endeavors?
3. What are your further learning goals?

GUIDELINES FOR TECHNOLOGY TEACHING STRATEGIES AND BUILDING THE LEARNING COMMUNITY

Quick Tips for Promoting the Learning Community

1. Acknowledge diverse learners. Recognize contributions of individuals and provide opportunities for individuals to participate in self-assessment and peer review.

2. Participate in the learning community, but don't dominate it. In the online setting, provide regular communications to affirm social presence.
3. Provide learning spaces for the community's work, including online discussions and document sharing. This can be in the form of online discussion boards, wiki spaces, or collaborative concept mapping tools.

Questions for Further Reflection

1. In designing activities for the learning community, what activities will best promote learning together about a topic?
2. While technology often helps us bring more diverse students to our classrooms, how do we most effectively meet our diverse students' needs in our courses?
3. What issues related to inappropriate use of technology need to be considered in course learning communities?

Learning Activity

1. Are there available social spaces that add to or challenge your work with students? Search a social space such as YouTube, a video sharing social space, on a topical area you currently teach or plan to teach.
2. Are there videos that might have relevance for sharing with one of your class learning communities? Are there videos you might steer your learning community away from?
3. What benefits and challenges do you identify in your nurse educator work with this type of social space?

Online Resources for Further Learning

- *Web 2.0 in Teaching and Learning*: http://net.educause.edu/ir/library/pdf/ERM0621.pdf
- *How to Share Bookmarks With People in Your del.icio.us Network*: http://www.ehow.com/how_2019685_sharing-bookmarks-delicious.html
- *Let's Face Facebook.* This brief article by M. Eodice and D. Gaffin discusses the pros and cons of Facebook: http://www.ou.edu/etc/medialib/university_college/Documents.Par.81233.File.dat/Eodice&Gaffin08.pdf

REFERENCES

Bain, K. (2004). *What the best college teachers do.* Cambridge, MA: Harvard University Press.

Brookfield, S., & Preskill, S. (2005). *Discussions as a way of teaching* (2nd ed.). San Francisco, CA: Jossey-Bass.

Carnegie Mellon University. (2009). *Enhancing education: Learning principles.* Retrieved October 16, 2009, from http://www.cmu.edu/teaching/principles/learning.html

Dufour, R., & Eaker, R. (1998). *Professional learning communities at work: Best practices for enhancing student achievement.* Bloomington, IN: Solution Tree Publishing.

Fink, L. D. (2003). *Creating significant learning experiences: An integrated approach to designing college courses.* San Francisco: Jossey-Bass.

Institute of Medicine. (2003). *Health professions education: A bridge to quality.* Washington, DC: National Academies Press.

International Society for Technology in Education. (2004). *The national educational technology standards and performance indicators for teachers.* Retrieved October 16, 2009, from http://www.iste.org/Content/NavigationMenu/NETS/ForTeachers/2008 Standards/NETS_T_Standards_Final.pdf

Kroen, K., & Bonnel, W. (2007, February). *Applied learning, group assignments and online courses: Toward developing best practices.* Conference on Applied Learning in Higher Education, St. Joseph, MO.

Michaelsen, L. K. (1998). *Three keys to using learning groups effectively.* The University of Oklahoma. Retrieved September 2, 2009, from http://www.med.wright.edu/aa/facdev/_Files/PDFfiles/ThreeKeys.pdf

Murray, H., Gillese, E., Lennon, M., Mercer, P., & Robinson, M. (1996). *American Association of Higher Education bulletin.* Retrieved October 16, 2009, from http://www.aahea.org/bulletins/articles/Ethical+Principles.htm

Oblinger, D. (2003). Boomers, GenXers, Millennials: Understanding the new students. *Educause Review, 38,* 37–47.

Palloff, R. M., & Pratt, K. (2004). *Collaborating online: Learning together in community.* San Francisco: Jossey-Bass.

Ribble, M., Bailey, G., & Ross, T. (2004). Digital citizenship, addressing appropriate technology behavior. *Learning and Leading with Technology, 32*(1), 6–11.

Sampson, E., & Marthas, M. (1990). *Group process for health profession.* Albany, NY: Delmar Publishing.

Skiba, D. (2005). The Millennials: Have they arrived at your school of nursing? *Nursing Education Perspectives, 26*(6), 370–371.

University of Sydney. (n.d). *Groupwork for staff, designing, assessing, and managing.* Retrieved September 2, 2009, from http://teaching.econ.usyd.edu.au/groupwork/WhyGroupwork/01a_why.html

Vella, J. (2002). *Learning to listen, learning to teach: The power of dialogue in educating adults.* San Francisco, CA: Jossey-Bass.

Wiggins, G., & McTighe, J. (1998). *Understanding by design.* Alexandria, VA: Association for Supervision & Curriculum Development.

Young, J. R. (2001, November 9). Does "digital divide" rhetoric do more harm than good? *The Chronicle of Higher Education,* A51.

8   Technologies and Active Learning

CHAPTER GOAL

Gain resources and strategies for making active learning an integral part of a teaching toolbox.

BEGINNING REFLECTION

1. What experiences have you had that relate to creating active learning assignments?
2. What ideas do you have for assignments for which you might incorporate active learning?

INTRODUCTION

Learning is complex in today's technology-rich world. Technology has made it much easier to deliver learning activities and assignments to students. Active learning with technologies provides students with the opportunity to integrate actual world experiences into virtual or face-to-face class experiences, truly experiencing course content. Technology can bring students opportunities for doing and learning in both actual and virtual worlds (Bonk, 2009).

This chapter is about making learning real and active, considering technology as a tool for promoting active learning. Appropriate for either traditional classroom teaching or online courses, technology-supported active learning assignments can be timely, efficient approaches for teaching and for enhancing student learning. Opportunity for creativity in using technology as a part of active learning assignments abounds. Fink (2003) noted that one of the most important things faculty can do to promote learning is expand active learning activities.

WHAT ARE ACTIVE LEARNING ASSIGNMENTS?

Assignments are considered any activities that help students learn or that assess student learning. These activities provide an opportunity to apply content for practice and learning (Fink, 2003). Assignments serve as tools to help students focus on concepts, helping them better understand and use new information in meaningful ways. Student skill sets are developed via well-designed assignments based on learning objectives.

Adult education theory (Knowles, 1984) posits that students learn by applying concepts in meaningful ways. Active learning engages students in doing something with the content that is being taught. Brookfield and Preskill (2005) describe the importance of engaging the body as well as the mind in learning. In contrast to more traditional lecture formats, faculty can engage students and extend students' knowledge of course content using varied technologies. In an active learning mode, students gain information, do something with the information, and then reflect on what has been learned. Students miss real world applications if they only sit and listen to classroom presentations or just read and answer basic factual study questions to complete online courses.

In nursing, a clinical practice component is an expected part of student learning. Our challenge with classroom teaching becomes helping students prepare for safe clinical practice. Doing something with specified content gives students practice in synthesizing knowledge and skills in preparation for the complex tasks they will be completing in clinical settings. When learning how to do otoscopic exams, for example, students can read about the topic and observe practitioners, but often it is not until they actively practice or apply the strategy in the clinical lab or with patients that the concepts make sense. While we want students to read and understand key information, it is more likely they will understand and recall the concepts if they apply the concepts via projects of some type. Often it is not until students are working on assigned projects that key points come together. Active learning strategies can range from discussion questions, to role playing, to virtual tours. Technology makes active learning tools—from flashcards to question and answer games or automated quizzes—all more accessible.

Active learning carries through the theme of helping students learn how to learn; students gain practice in active situations that will help them transition to practice. Students gain skills for lifelong learning as well. Various concepts related to active learning have related or similar meanings. The terms *active learning, authentic learning, applied learning,* and *experiential learning* are often used in close association. Each term describes opportunities for students to apply knowledge and skills in an immediate and relevant setting (Knowles, 1984). For our purposes, we will use the following broad descriptors.

- **Active learning.** *Active learning* will be considered the broader term in this discussion. It refers to using or doing something with information gained. Information would be gained from a reading, for example, and then applied via some type of activity or assignment. Active learning makes the connection between the facts presented and actual clinical application (Fink, 2003).
- **Authentic learning.** Authentic learning occurs when active strategies are used to engage in realistic activities or develop projects with relevance to a real need.
- **Applied learning.** Applied learning is beneficial in reminding us to take information gained in the classroom to the clinical or community setting (a common approach in health professions education).
- **Experiential learning.** Experiential learning is considered learning around experiences including direct participation in specific activities. Students reflect and gain meaning.

Teaching approaches are used in each context that make learning real and active to meet diverse learner needs. Within each approach, students gain the opportunity to be more engaged in learning. For the purposes of our discussion, terms will be grouped under the concepts of active learning. Technology provides opportunities to make teaching and learning more active.

WHAT ARE BEST PRACTICES RELATED TO ACTIVE LEARNING?

Active learning is consistent with a variety of theories and best practices. Examples include the following:

- **Adult learning theory** (Knowles, 1984). Adult learning theory reminds us to ask, when developing lesson plans, how we can build on students' current knowledge/experience, make the content relevant to students, and help them apply that content.
- **Constructivist learning theory** (Savery & Duffy, 1995). Constructivism reminds us to provide assignments that are useful to students in constructing their own learning and understanding.
- **Principles for good practices in teaching.** Chickering and Gamson's (1987) seven research-supported principles for undergraduate education include a focus on using active learning techniques that respect diverse learners' talents and ways of learning.
- **Principles of learning.** Carnegie Mellon University (2009) shares research-supported learning principles, consistent with active learning, that include building on content learning, combining and integrating content with practice, and understanding when to apply content learned.

TECHNOLOGY AND ACTIVE LEARNING: AUDIO AND VISUAL EXAMPLES

Whether our teaching is online, face-to-face, or in a clinical setting, a key concept includes making a good fit between the learning we want for students and the assignments and technology tools that we choose for our classes. Providing students with a variety of assignment types helps meet the needs of diverse learners. While listening to an audio presentation or watching a video provides learning opportunities, these activities are often completed while doing something else or multitasking. Technology provides opportunities to engage diverse learners who bring diverse learning styles to class. Visual, auditory, and kinesthetic learning styles can all be enhanced by a variety of technology-supported assignments.

Active Auditory Learning

Listening has long been a component of learning. Intonation is part of our language and provides cues to meaning. We use verbal cues in many ways in the classroom, such as accepting and reacting to student emotions, providing positive reinforcement, giving appropriate classroom feedback to students, using questioning as a tool, giving information, and giving direction. We also use nonverbal cues in the classroom, such as eye contact, gestures, mannerisms, movement, facial expressions, posture, energy level, and use of space. When audio becomes the focus, the educator is challenged to make the audio presentation to the point, interesting, and engaging.

In the authors' early graduate school years, listening to audio tapes while driving seemed a good use of time. MP3 players such as iPods have since taken their place and bring even more flexibility to learning on the run. Podcasts have made learning on the go a popular feature highlighting interest in audio learning. Faculty are creating podcasts of lectures and delivering these to students via a school-specific version of the iTunes University store (http://www.apple.com/education/guidedtours/itunesu. html). How best to use audio in our teaching and learning is an important concept for further discussion (Fleming, 2009).

Additionally, tools including voice-over PowerPoint presentations and classroom capture tools such as Camtasia expand and provide enhanced audio learning opportunities. Tools such as Elluminate add an interactive component to audio learning as well. While these technologies provide teaching/learning opportunities, best practices need to be considered in their implementation.

How can audio be used as active learning? The Podcast Group (http://www.podcast.net/) suggests that faculty listen to a 30-minute podcast, and then ask three questions:

- How much of the material did I retain?
- Did I focus the entire time on the podcast (or was I multitasking in a way that prevented engaging in the learning)?
- What other ways do I think the content might have been presented to better engage the learner?

As noted, asking learners to do something with the information helps keep them engaged. This strategy can be as basic as asking learners to complete a worksheet based on the audio session or reflecting on specified questions.

Active Visual or Video Learning

Visual images can help convey key points and place learning in context. For example, simple diagrams can help students recall complex anatomy or physiology concepts and more easily place content in context. Visual learners in particular benefit from a variety of visual learning tools such as flowcharts, graphs, and colors (Fleming, 2009).

Videos bring additional visual learning opportunities. Benefits to using videos include convenience issues for students, the potential for active learning when used correctly, benefits of "demonstrating" content, accessing "real-life" cases/interviews; and the potential for "re-runs/ reviews" that can benefit the student. For many videos, just being able to stop and start the video at convenient times allows opportunity to discuss topics in class or to "replay" key points.

Videos also make us observers and can serve many purposes in teaching and learning. Often in health care, videos benefit by depicting very personal situations or critical care situations that it would be hard for large student numbers to observe in real time. For example, providing a video tour of the operating room before clinical experiences may promote an easier transition to this setting and make the tour accessible to increased numbers of students. Faculty play important roles in setting the learning stage for video and debriefing the experience, whether face-to-face or online.

Concepts and boundaries of video are blurring. Videos are shown in face-to-face classrooms, on computer-based DVDs, or as Web-based scenarios. Video applications have recently included streaming video (video on the Internet); instructional televised video in the classroom via a two-way interactive connection; one-way live video to the classroom with opportunity for call-in questions; and compact disc–based videos (CD-ROM). Video for the traditional classroom, such as resources from the Public Broadcasting System, are available as well.

Faculty roles with a video presentation include much more than just "plugging it in." The same teaching learning concepts of engaging students apply across a variety of video types. Relevant to active learning, we ask students to do something with the video content. For example, faculty might provide students discussion prompts or questions related to the video for students to think about while watching the video.

While our discussion does not relate to major video production, broad guidelines can help avoid "talking heads" or the "snooze factor" that prevail in some videos. Further tips for audiovisual teaching and learning are provided by the University of Idaho, Engineering Outreach (Willis, 2004). If you are assigning a specific audio or video activity, sample tips for engaging students for audio-video learning (synchronous or asynchronous) include:

- Orient or prepare students for what's going to be happening (create set either verbally or by written notation).
- Incorporate active learning (some strategy for interacting with the video content such as questions to answer or work sheets as a pre-post activity).
- Provide opportunities to discuss and debrief the learning points from the video.

If you are presenting content via a video presentation:

- Avoid being a "talking head." Incorporate engaging prompts or questions for student reflection.
- Be prepared for presentations in order to avoid the distraction of shuffled papers.
- Be aware of your nonverbal motions and consider if these distract from the message (completing a self-assessment on a video of your own teaching can be useful).

Challenges in Audiovisual Learning

While there are many benefits in audiovisual learning, there are also challenges to consider. What are our roles as providers of audiovisual materials, for example with the following issues?

- Great variability exists in the quality of audio and video materials available. What is our faculty role in the critique of these tools before sharing them with students?
- What is the faculty role in production? Should faculty create videos? How professional do these videos need to be? What resources are available? Does something available already capture the desired teaching concepts? A fair amount of time, energy, and resources go into completing a professional quality video. It is also harder to make changes to a video than to a Web page.
- What are the issues when students seek their own online videos as learning tools? What types of review criteria should students have for choosing online videos to watch?
- What are the benefits and challenges of assignments where students create their own videos?

ACTIVE LEARNING MODES: AUTHENTIC ASSIGNMENTS

Putting learning into context, whether online or face-to-face, is an important faculty role. Isolated facts are easily forgotten, and context created by faculty helps students make sense of factual information. Strategies for expanding our toolbox of active learning strategies fall into the following broad categories: Stories, Cases, Interviews, and Observations. Even though we are using technologies, we are back to the basics of familiar tools/concepts and good educational principles.

Stories and Cases

Stories and cases are closely related concepts, with stories providing a more descriptive, narrative approach and cases a more detailed factual approach. Both provide opportunities to share examples in a nonthreatening way that promotes opportunity for thought and discussion. These tools can provide either an introduction to or a reinforcement of a topic area. Stories can bring a more humanistic component to teaching with technologies. Stories and cases help faculty accomplish the following goals:

- Provide the connection between the textbook and the lived experience, making concepts more easily memorable.
- Relate new concepts to other more familiar concepts.
- Show how concepts can be applied in similar ways across different populations or settings, extending understandings about certain illnesses. For example a scenario could be provided of two different patients, one with early Parkinson's disease and one with late-stage Parkinson's disease.

Problem-based learning, incorporating the concept of ongoing expanding stories or cases, is another related concept with benefits of case sharing. Today's technologies allow stories to be shared in new and important ways, as described at chapter end in the "Evidence-Based Review Abstract: Storytelling as a Teaching and Learning Concept."

Interview and Observation Assignments

Authentic assignments that engage students with real world experiences provide another opportunity for expanding learning with technology. These authentic assignments provide students opportunities to learn from experts on selected topics and gain real world perspectives. Student reflections and summaries can be shared with the learning community to extend perspectives on a topic. Completing interview assignments with professionals working in a specialty clinical area, for example, students can learn and gain from these experts. This activity also provides students opportunities to seek and gain mentors.

Developing observation assignments for students, whether direct observation or participant observation, provides students opportunity to add real world perspective to class concepts. Students learning about group theory, for example, might observe a community-based group education session or support group. Further ideas for engaging students with interviews and observations are provided by Bonnel and Meek (2007).

CREATING MEANINGFUL ASSIGNMENTS

All assignments are not created equal. What makes one assignment better than another? How do we creatively put together interesting learning activities for our students? Rather than asking "What should I cover in this class?" asking "What should my students learn to do?" provides more direction. Walvoord and Anderson (1998) describe concepts of fit and feasibility in assignment design. Focusing on the "doing" component of learning can guide assignment development.

Particularly with text-based communication, we want clear, accessible guidelines. These guidelines include being clear as to whether the assignment is for supporting ongoing learning or serves as part of a final grade. The concepts of formative and summative evaluation are discussed further in Chapter 9. Developing a course assignment map of when and where assignments exist in the semester can be useful (Walvoord & Anderson, 1998). This approach also helps to see whether assignments fit course goals and whether these assignments are manageable in terms of workload. This map helps develop an assignment-centered course with focus on outcomes rather than content. Building on concepts within the Integrated Learning Triangle for Teaching With Technologies (Appendix B) provides direction. Sample points to consider in writing an assignment include:

- Consider the context. What is the context for this assignment? Who are the students? What type of course will this assignment be incorporated into?

- Include a strong purpose statement. What is the point of this assignment? How will completing this assignment help students prepare for current or future practice? How will this activity help students learn? Including an assignment introduction helps students understand the major intent of the assignment and lets them know what's in it for them.
- Determine your objectives for the assignment. Specific assignment objectives lay the framework for assignment evaluation. Questions to guide objectives development include the following: What is the point of this assignment? How will this activity help students engage in active learning? How does this activity help students improve their critical thinking?
- Use activities that actively engage students with using the content. As noted earlier, active engagement promotes students in learning and promotes critical thinking.
- Name assignments to help convey the intended learning goals. A good assignment name used consistently also helps avoid confusion when communicating with students.
- Provide clear directions. Particularly with text-based communication that lacks immediate opportunities for clarification, potential for student confusion in reading directions exists. While our guidelines can seem fairly clear to us, usually we can benefit from having additional readers give feedback as to clarity of the guidelines. Alfaro-LeFevre (2001) provides further discussion on assignment development.

Reflection as Added Value for Assignments

Self-reflection provides additional opportunity for interaction with the content. As students reflect on an assignment, they gain an opportunity to build on their past experiences and incorporate current learning experiences. Whether online or in-class, Fink (2003) has noted that one relatively easy way to both engage students and extend learning includes asking our students to complete more self-reflections.

For example, self-reflection against an assignment rubric helps students gain skills in judging the quality of their work, judging their self-knowledge, and determining when more learning is needed. Billings (2005) noted that self-reflection helps students learn how to transfer concepts from theory to practice and from one context to another. Reflection provides an opportunity to think about learning from one's experience and leads to self-directed learning. Providing benchmark indicators via rubrics and asking students to identify how they have accomplished these helps gain student perceptions of outcomes.

Assignment Repositories

Many electronic repositories are being developed of useful resources and assignments for teaching students across a variety of settings. These sites for gathering electronic documents and resources for teaching/learning provide a win-win situation, often providing active learning assignment ideas for faculty. The Quality & Safety Education for Nurses (QSEN) repository, for example, focuses on resources and assignments that can be used to help students gain recommended Health Professions Educator competencies. Opportunities exist for others to use these assignments, further evaluate them, and then share them with others. Peer review opportunities exist as part of many of these repositories to assist in further developing best teaching strategies. They also serve as an opportunity for peer review to promote scholarship with our teaching. Sample resources are provided in Exhibit 8.1.

Additionally, student textbooks often have accompanying faculty and student guides either in electronic or hard copy format. While these resources vary in depth, many of the assignment suggestions can easily be adapted to fit specific course needs and technologies.

Exhibit 8.1

ELECTRONIC REPOSITORIES

Sample repositories providing resources for active learning assignments can be found at the following Web sites.

- Quality & Safety Education for Nurses (QSEN) resources, http://www.qsen.org
- Multimedia Educational Resource for Learning and Online Teaching, http://www.merlot.org/merlot/index.htm
- World Lecture Hall, http://web.austin.utexas.edu/wlh/
- MIT OpenCourseWare, http://ocw.mit.edu
- MedEdPORTAL, www.aamc.org/mededportal
- Learning Objects, Learning Exchange, http://www.lolaexchange.org/
- The Health Education Assets Library (HEAL), http://www.healcentral.org/

Exhibit 8.2

EVIDENCE-BASED REVIEW ABSTRACT: STORYTELLING AS A TEACHING AND LEARNING CONCEPT

Compiled by: Cheryl Spittler, MS, RN, CEN, CPSN

Storytelling has been around since the beginning of time and is a way to learn history, communicate information, and can be viewed as a form of entertainment. It is a familiar way of relating information and can provide knowledge on different topics. A systematic literature review identified that both qualitative and quantitative researchers have found that evidence-based practice exists for storytelling. Storytelling is an inexpensive teaching method and can be used to understand the meaning of an experience and improve the process of learning. Possible benefits of telling a story are to express information uniquely, aid in problem solving, provide diversity in the ways of knowing, make learning more memorable, and contribute to another way of knowing. In regards to patient education, stories may help people gain confidence with procedures, acquire skills quicker, decrease stress, aid in patient/family trust development, and improve memory retention.

Additionally, storytelling may lead to further truths on different topics and help patients understand the meaning of experiences in a better way. A model case was developed of storytelling as a teaching and learning concept for use with a group of women diagnosed with breast cancer. Listening to podcasts with other cancer survivor testimonies is a way to use storytelling to convey important information such as treatment options and decisions, personal experiences, frequently encountered problems and concerns, and knowing how to access available support services. Technology serves as a tool for conveying the stories. Further research specific to combining storytelling with technologies is recommended.

Bibliography

Bronwynne, C. E., & Crogan, N. L. (2008). Storytelling intervention of patients with cancer: Part I development and implementation. *Oncology Nursing Forum, 35*(2), 257–264.

Cangelosi, P. R., & Whitt, K. J. (2006). Teaching through storytelling: An exemplar. *International Journal of Nursing Education Scholarship, 3*(1). Retrieved June 18, 2008, from http://www.bepress.com/ijnes/vol3/iss1/art2/

Carter, B. (2007). Good and bad stories: Decisive moments, shock and awe and being moral. *Journal of Clinical Nursing, 17*(8), 1063–1070.

Crogan, N. L., & Bronwynne, C. E. (2008). Storytelling intervention for patients with cancer: Part 2—Pilot testing. *Oncology Nursing Forum, 35*(2), 265–272.

Davidhizar, R., & Lonser, G. (2003). Story-telling as a teaching technique. *Nurse Educator, 28*(5), 217–221.

Gere, J., Kozlovich, B., & Kelin, D. A. (2002). *By word of mouth: A storytelling guide for the classroom.* Retrieved June 18, 2008, from http://www.prel.org/products/pr_/storytelling.htm

Giddens, J. F. (2007). The neighborhood: A web-based platform to support conceptual teaching and learning. *Nursing Education Perspectives, 28*(5), 251–256.

Giddens, J. F. (2008). Achieving diversity in nursing through multicontextual learning environments. *Nursing Outlook, 56*(2), 78–83.

(Continued)

Exhibit 8.2

EVIDENCE-BASED REVIEW ABSTRACT: STORYTELLING AS A TEACHING AND LEARNING CONCEPT (*Continued*)

Hsieh, W., Smith, B. K., & Stefanou, S. P. (2004). *It is more about telling interesting stories: Use explicit hints in storytelling to help college students solve ill-defined problems.* Retrieved September 30, 2009, from http://eric.ed.gov/ERICWebPortal/recordDetail?accno=ED485034

Lordly, D. (2007). Once upon a time . . . Story-telling to enhance teaching and learning. *Canadian Journal of Dietetic Practice and Research, 68*(1), 30–35.

Milton, C. L. (2006). Fables: Ways of knowing and understanding the meaning in nursing. *Nursing Science Quarterly, 19*(2), 100–103.

Wallace-Banks, J. (2002). Talk that talk: Story-telling and analysis rooted in African American oral tradition. *Qualitative Health Research, 12*(3), 410–426.

As discussed previously in the chapter, the evidence-based review abstract "Storytelling as a Teaching and Learning Concept" is provided in Exhibit 8.2. This synthesis of best evidence provides further direction for our work as educators.

SUMMARY

Technology provides an opportunity to increase active learning for our students, making learning real and authentic. The types of learning activities we provide help students gain skills for their future professional practice. The report on Health Professions Education (Institute of Medicine, 2003) includes incorporating technology into curricula as one of its top five priority competencies. A variety of assignments helps meet students' diverse learning needs and prepare students for practice. Active learning, including audio and visual learning modes, as well as authentic assignments such as interviews and observations, provides tools for engaging students for learning.

ENDING REFLECTION

1. What is the most important content that you learned in this chapter?
2. What are your plans for using the information in this chapter in your future teaching endeavors?
3. What are your further learning goals?

GUIDELINES FOR TECHNOLOGIES AND ACTIVE LEARNING

Quick Tips to Promote Active Learning

1. Use a variety of technology-based mediums, such as audio, video, and applied learning to meet diverse learners' needs.
2. Provide relevant student assignments with clear purpose statements and guidelines.
3. Provide opportunities for learners to share their stories (or experiences) and build on these stories in teaching sessions.

Questions for Further Reflection

1. What ways can audiovisuals be presented to best engage our students?
2. What are benefits and challenges of synchronous versus asynchronous uses of audiovisual learning?
3. In what ways can audiovisual materials help extend meaningful faculty presence?

Learning Activity: Technology Interview

Select someone in your nursing school or health care agency who has experience teaching with a selected technology. Ask this individual if "in the spirit of knowledge sharing" he or she would be willing to talk with you about his or her experiences teaching with a particular technology. Sample questions might include the following:

1. What types of students and courses do you use this technology with?
2. What do you like about teaching with this technology?
3. Is there a particular assignment you like for engaging students and promoting active learning?
4. What were some of the challenges for you in getting started teaching with this technology? What have been some of the positive outcomes you have seen?
5. What advice do you have for a new faculty member beginning work in teaching with this particular technology?

Online Resources for Further Learning

■ Critical Thinking, Key Concepts (select from the Library/Articles section). This resource provides further review and teaching tips for developing critical thinking from the Center for Critical Thinking: www.criticalthinking.org

■ Teaching Tools and Techniques, Techniques for Student Engagement and Classroom Management in Large (and Small) Classes. This resource on engaging students is provided by the National Teaching and Learning Forum: http://www.ntlf.com/html/lib/sup pmat/teachingtools.pdf

REFERENCES

Alfaro-LeFevre, R. (2001). Thinking critically about your assignments. *Nurse Educator* 26(1), 15–16.

Billings, D. (2005). Teaching for higher order learning. *Journal of Continuing Education in Nursing, 36*(6), 244–245.

Bonk, C. (2009). *The world is open: How Web technology is revolutionizing education.* San Francisco: Jossey-Bass.

Bonnel, W., & Meek, V. (2007). Qualitative assignments to enhance online learning communities. *Instructional Technology and Distance Learning, 4*(2), 49–54.

Brookfield, S. D., & Preskill, S. (2005). *Discussions as a way of teaching* (2nd ed.). San Francisco: Jossey-Bass.

Carnegie Mellon University. (2009). *Enhancing education: Learning principles.* Retrieved from http://www.cmu.edu/teaching/principles/learning.html

Chickering, A. W., & Gamson, A. F. (1987). *Seven principles for good practice in undergraduate education.* Retrieved October 16, 2009, from http://honolulu.hawaii.edu/intranet/committees/FacDevCom/guidebk/teachtip/7princip.htm

Fink, L. D. (2003). *Creating significant learning experiences: An integrated approach to designing college courses.* San Francisco: Jossey-Bass.

Fleming, N. (2009). *VARK, a guide to learning styles.* Retrieved October 16, 2009, from http://www.vark-learn.com/english/index.asp

Institute of Medicine. (2003). *Health professions education: A bridge to quality.* Washington, DC: National Academies Press.

Knowles, M. (1984). *The adult learner: A neglected species.* Houston, TX: Gulf Publishing.

Savery, J., & Duffy, T. (1995). Problem based learning: An instructional model and its constructivist framework. *Educational Technology, 35*, 31–38.

Walvoord, B., & Anderson, V. (1998). *Effective grading: A tool for learning and assessment.* San Francisco: Jossey-Bass.

Willis, B. (2004). *Distance education at a glance.* Retrieved from http://www.uiweb.uidaho.edu/eo/dist5.html

9 Feedback, Debriefing, and Evaluation With Technology

CHAPTER GOAL

Gain perspective on the technological options for teaching and evaluating student achievement.

BEGINNING REFLECTION

1. What experiences have you had giving feedback to students?
2. With what evaluation techniques are you most familiar and comfortable?
3. How can technology promote reasonable and effective evaluations?

INTRODUCTION

The public needs to have confidence that students and graduates in the health professions are safe practitioners. This chapter discusses the use of a variety of technologies to evaluate and provide feedback to students. Technology and evaluation are a good match, with technology providing many flexible options for assessment, evaluation, and feedback. Technology can help faculty be fair and consistent. Evaluation is an essential part of the planning process for both courses and assignments. Effective grading involves assignments that fit learning goals (Walvoord & Anderson, 1998). Broad principles of good evaluation developed by the American Association of Higher Education Assessment Forum (1993) provide background for this chapter discussion.

Learning management systems and audience response systems (clickers), for example, often provide opportunities for instant testing with immediate feedback that can promote learning. The concepts of feedback and evaluation are considered broadly in this chapter as learning tools. Evaluation can be both simple and complex. The expectation is to compare student performance with expected outcomes. The reality is that numerous factors can interfere with that comparison. Our goal is to evaluate student knowledge rather than student stress levels. While a focus on grades is an inherent part of the educational system and can be a powerful student motivator, a focus only on grades is less likely to encourage a mindset for lifelong learning. Helping students and student groups gain a vision for success is more likely to encourage students toward lifelong learning.

Teaching, learning, and evaluation concepts create a cyclic process and build on each other. Building on assessed needs, new content is typically presented for learning. Students are subsequently evaluated to determine the extent to which goals/objectives for the acquisition of new content were met. The most effective evaluation then becomes a teaching tool to help students with additional learning or to reinforce what has already been learned. Feedback is the process by which students gain information about their performance on the evaluation measures. Additionally, evaluation in nursing education is best considered as part of a systematic approach that integrates evaluation across classroom, clinical lab, and clinical experiences. Theory application is tested in the classroom; safety competencies are checked off in the learning lab; application with actual patients is gained in the clinical setting.

Why is this topic essential in a book about teaching with technology? First, the explosion of new technologies offers continuously new ways to assess and evaluate students and to provide feedback, so faculty need to know the options and make considered decisions about which to use. Faculty must also be cognizant of the sensitive nature of feedback, especially in a technology-rich world. Sometimes the feedback students must be given is not positive, and faculty need to choose the best and most responsible mechanisms by which to relay this information. As faculty, we remember that many technological methods, while fast and accessible, are impersonal at best (recall Shea's [1994] rules of netiquette). As a result, certain technologies make it harder for faculty to soften any negative feedback or determine how students are interpreting and responding to that feedback. More scholarship is needed for establishing best practices on providing feedback through text-based media.

EVALUATION AND ITS RELATIONSHIP TO TEACHING

Assessment, Feedback, and Evaluation

There are a number of related terms—assessment, feedback, and evaluation—that are often confused or used without regard for their subtle differences. Assessment is the process used to "gather, summarize, interpret, and use data to decide a direction for action" (Bastable, 2008, pp. 559–560). Feedback builds on assessment. Feedback has been described as information communicated to students that is based on an assessment and that helps the student reflect and work further with the information provided. This includes constructing self-knowledge relevant to course learning and setting further learning goals (Bonnel, Ludwig, & Smith, 2007). Feedback is usually most effective when it is as timely and objective as possible.

Building on both assessment and feedback, evaluation is the process used to "gather, summarize, interpret, and use data to determine the extent to which an action was successful" (Bastable, 2008, p. 560). While assessment-based feedback provides direction for actions, evaluation implies a final judgment about the success of actions. Because of this fundamental difference, assessment and feedback are commonly conducted early in the semester and continue in an ongoing fashion throughout the teaching/learning process (to guide further teaching/learning). Evaluation is often conducted later in the semester or process (to establish goal/objective achievement). Evaluation frequently occurs through formal grades but can occur through ongoing informal mechanisms as well.

Norm Referenced and Criteria Referenced

Another perspective divides evaluation into norm referenced and criterion referenced. Norm-referenced evaluation compares any given learner with other students or groups of students (either a standardized group or the student's fellow classmates), while criterion-referenced evaluation compares the learner with an objective set of criteria. Usually, in norm-referenced evaluations, faculty seek a predetermined distribution of grades that fits a bell curve, with a few students getting very high and very low grades and most students earning average grades. Grading on this curve can be challenging, in that it minimizes faculty opportunities to evaluate student competency against pre-set criteria (Ericksen, 2008). Criterion-referenced evaluation relates to meeting a criterion and does not generally have a predetermined grade distribution. In fact, if all students meet the set of criteria, then all students pass the evaluation; if no student meets the set criteria, then no one passes.

Formative and Summative Evaluation

The process of evaluation is further defined as formative or summative. Formative evaluation is similar to feedback in general and is part of the ongoing learning process. Formative evaluation is conducted during the teaching/learning process to help identify strengths and weaknesses and further guide learning activities. Formative evaluation, therefore, and assessment are very similar in nature and may, at times, overlap with one another. Periodic formative evaluations help shape students into the proficient nurses they want to be. Summative evaluation, on the other hand, implies a final summary of learning and reflects the more conventional view of evaluation that occurs at the end of the teaching/learning process to determine if objectives/goals were met and to what extent they were met. The evaluation determines if students have met the criteria to be that proficient nurse. Summative evaluation has been described as "taking assessment to the next level where judgments are made about the value/quality of performance at some endpoint" (Billings & Halstead, 2009, p. 409).

Assessment and Teaching With Technology

Technology provides multiple opportunities for enhancing assessment of student learning and for providing feedback to students. Assessment can be completed before starting to teach (a lesson, or a course, or a lab procedure) to see what knowledge students bring with them to the teaching situation. Ongoing assessments, or formative evaluations, may be conducted to determine students' learning to date, identify problems, and help guide the teaching process.

At the beginning of a course or individual class, students can be assessed for their current knowledge level. This assessment may consist of a timed multiple choice test in which the testing option closes after just 5 or 10 minutes (faculty determined), or it may consist of small group discussion following questions based on the day's required readings. Both of these options could also be used to conduct formative evaluation as the semester proceeds, or an informal, low-stakes writing exercise during class might provide formative feedback. Summative evaluation may consist of a timed, open book examination that occurs synchronously for all students, or it may consist of a more formal, high-stakes writing assignment, or a formal presentation that is transmitted to the entire class via the video network or Wimba, a type of collaborative learning software.

Almost inevitably in a formal course, some type of summative evaluation will occur to determine students' final achievement (or lack thereof) of the learning goals and objectives. Under the best of circumstances that evaluation then becomes a teaching tool from which students further cement their learning of content and skills.

Assessment and Remediation

Diverse learning needs and learning styles bring challenges to all classrooms, with the potential need for remediation in selected areas. Remediation, considered a remedy or attempt to improve limited skills, allows students an opportunity to correct errors or deficiencies in needed knowledge. For example, a number of educational testing companies, such as Assessment Technologies Institute (ATI), Health Education Systems, Incorporated (HESI), and Kaplan, offer an array of standardized assessments. Many are based on the concept that students must assess their current knowledge base in order to identify their achievement to date, and then also gain a focused study plan that they can adapt to their own unique knowledge deficits, learning style, and needs. Such standardized assessments offer review, practice, and guidance in weak areas. Remediation is consistent with goal setting and contracting for improved skill sets. As a part of formative evaluation, students can then enhance their abilities to do well on subsequent summative evaluations.

THE MANY FORMS OF FEEDBACK

Feedback is the general term for providing students information about their performance, and technology helps with that process, whether the goal is assessment, formative evaluation, summative evaluation, or even remediation. Technology provides many options (with more being discovered every day), often with advantages in efficiency and effectiveness over more traditional evaluation methods. Online quizzes, for example, provide opportunities for multiple reviews. High-fidelity simulations provide technological options in a safe environment in which students can learn new skills (which were formerly learned on real patients).

Also, technologies tend to provide hands-on experience that fit the theoretical principles of active learning discussed in an earlier chapter. Technological options also provide a means to ensure that all students have the same, required experiences. For example, if all students in an obstetrics course need to demonstrate the competency of assisting with the delivery of a baby, they all can meet this requirement using simulation; if all students in a critical care course need to provide CPR, now they all can. Sample options for using technology in self-assessment/reflection, peer evaluation, rubrics, and debriefing follow.

Self-Assessment and Student Reflection

While faculty have often been the major source of feedback, there is great value in feedback received from one's own experience and that of peers. Self-assessment based on self-reflection serves many purposes, but, among the most important, it establishes the students' role in and responsibility for their own learning. As students assess their own learning gains or deficits, learning that has already occurred can be strengthened or extended as students identify areas for continued growth and learning.

Honest self-reflection can prepare students to be open to feedback from others and to integrate that feedback into their own, self-directed learning. Self-assessment becomes self-evaluation when students judge their performance in comparison to objective criteria. Where there are gaps, self-assessment can help set the path for further learning. Self-assessment provides faculty a window into students' thinking (Driscoll & Wood, 2007). Fink (2003) noted that it is critical to learn to self-assess in order to prepare for the future, making this skill an important one for lifelong learning.

In addition to more traditional student evaluation methods, student self-assessment is a common approach to assess and document student learning. Students can be asked in all courses, for example, to complete pre- and postcourse self-assessments against course objectives. In addition to promoting student engagement in the course, this strategy also provides faculty information about student perspectives on status and performance and helps faculty provide better student feedback. An evidence-based review abstract, "Reflective Journaling," is shared at chapter end. This systematic review provides faculty direction for developing reflective assignments for students' clinical activities.

Peer Evaluation

Peer evaluation is an important tool by which students learn skills for the future. Peer review will be an important part of students' roles on clinical teams. Benefits of peer evaluation include learning opportunities and exchange in sharing feedback with others. Criteria to promote fair peer evaluation include clear standards and guides and explain the professional role of the evaluator. Given the proper guidance, students can use peer evaluation to provide meaningful feedback. Whether peers are fellow students or fellow clinical staff, it is critical that they be given clear evaluation guidelines and that they evaluate only content or skills that they are prepared to evaluate. Thus, effective orientation to this skill is important. Orientation includes not just what students will be doing, but why they will be doing it. Peer evaluation promotes the concept of professional responsibility and it helps develop the collaborative skills required to work effectively in teams. Peer feedback is also a needed lifelong skill.

As with all forms of evaluation, the primary challenge to effective self-assessment and peer evaluation is the potential for bias. The essential element is honesty and, when honesty is present, self- and peer feedback are helpful to both students and faculty. Sometimes students may be too hard on themselves or too easy on their peers (though the opposite can also be true).

Rubrics

Rubrics are developed to grade an assignment (either formative or summative), as well as to provide students guidance in assignment completion. These are good evaluation tools for many reasons. A rubric is an explicit summary, often in list form, of essential criteria for a project, with rating potential for each criterion. Faculty use of rubrics can promote timely, detailed feedback responses, encourage critical thinking, and facilitate student–faculty communication (Stevens & Levi, 2005). They have the benefit of providing more detailed information than one specific letter grade alone.

Rubrics can vary from simple to complex. A simple rubric for a writing assignment, for example, might include basic criteria for content, organization, and presentation (Tierney & Simon, 2004). Good rubrics can help students focus on what is important to learn rather than treating all facts as equally important. Rubrics provide both a learning tool and an evaluation tool. They are also beneficial for self-assessment and student peer

Exhibit 9.1

SAMPLE DEBRIEFING QUESTIONS

- How do you think the experience went?
- What were some of your successes?
- What were some of your failures?
- How was the team performance?

review. Rubrics provide students a guide for learning and project development and so serve as tools to teach self-directed learning. Providing rubrics at the initiation of an assignment gives students better direction on assignment expectations. Faculty can find these tools make grading easier and more consistent.

Debriefing as a Type of Feedback

Debriefing also provides an opportunity for feedback. Following a clinical experience, for example, it provides (often in a group setting) the opportunity to assess what happened, compare this to accepted criteria, and consider what worked or did not work. An important component of debriefing is asking students to engage in further goal setting or addressing what learning is still needed. The feedback or debriefing is lacking if further goal setting is not accomplished. Exhibit 9.1 provides sample debriefing questions.

SELECTED TECHNOLOGIES AND EVALUATION AND FEEDBACK

Classroom Response Systems (Clickers)

Clickers consist of both classroom hardware and software that connect the students, faculty, and audiovisual media. Students have small handheld devices that enable them to express their answers or views anonymously to other students in the classroom in aggregate form. The anonymous feature allows all students to participate, whether in a large class that would otherwise prohibit participation of all students or in a smaller class with students reluctant to express their individual views. Some automated-response programs offer faculty the ability to track individual student responses.

Clickers have the added benefit of providing immediate feedback to students and faculty so they can identify areas for additional time and attention. Clickers can be used at the beginning of class as a pre-assessment or to assess students' understanding of assigned readings. They can be used throughout a class period to provide ongoing feedback for students and faculty. Clickers can also be used as an evaluation technique at the end of a class period, with the advantage of providing virtually instantaneous feedback.

Learning Management Systems

Whether in a face-to-face course or an online course, computer-based classroom management systems are fast becoming the norm. While these systems provide a mechanism by which to organize course content (and computer links) and make it available to students at their convenience, they also provide multiple opportunities for teaching, learning, and evaluation (hence the term learning, rather than classroom, management systems). These systems provide a mechanism by which students can take exams (timed or not) and participate in online discussions (both synchronous and asynchronous). Grades can be posted so that students have access to their ongoing grade status. These systems allow short diagnostic and practice quizzes that help identify the strengths and weaknesses of students' knowledge base (Ericksen, 2008). While testing is just one aspect of evaluation, it is an important one because of its often high-stakes nature. If testing is the evaluation tool used, test questions need to be aligned with course goals (Driscoll & Wood, 2007; Fink, 2003). For example, if the lesson goal is critical thinking and just memorized information is tested, the test is not well aligned with teaching/learning goals.

Learning management systems provide item analysis opportunities to review test item performance. They provide opportunities to seek reliability and validity in the objective tests we as faculty implement. Many technologies are now available to promote easy review with an item analysis. Additional detail can often be gained from add-on programs. Technology provides the opportunity to make testing more reliable and valid, which, in a high-stakes testing situation, helps ensure fair testing. Item analysis becomes much easier with tools provided by learning management systems or added packages to review computer-based testing.

Standardized Computer Testing as a Learning Tool

Testing has also been described as a tool for instruction (Ericksen, 2008). Whether for actual testing situations or practice testing, computerized testing programs provide further learning opportunities. In nursing, for example, online testing programs such as Assessment Technologies Institute (ATI) and Kaplan provide the opportunity for students to participate in self-directed learning assessments. These practice tests can help prepare students for safe, knowledgeable practice as outlined by national boards.

This approach is different than testing in which students earn a grade but do not clearly understand what areas they are not performing well. Auto-mated practice tests can provide students immediate feedback on individual answers. Students gain benchmarks in matching their scores to others. If properly oriented, students can gain benefits of knowing where their weaknesses are and what learning areas they need to focus on. Additionally, students gain individualized learning plans with areas of study outlined.

Simulations

High-fidelity patient simulation (HFPS) provides multiple options for assessing, evaluating, and remediating content. For example, faculty might teach and/or assess current student knowledge by walking students through a scenario as it unfolds step by step. This process helps students integrate information and witness the faculty's rationale for decisions, as well as observe the patient's (HFPS) response to the actions taken. This approach might be appropriate for very new or very complicated content. Formative evaluation might consist of placing students in a scenario and letting it unfold naturally, according to the decisions (appropriate or not) that the students make and implement. For example, place students in a scenario where the patient (HFPS) unexpectedly codes and watch how the scenario unfolds. The use of rubrics for the experience would provide students rapid feedback on the quality of their performance, and that same rubric could be used for the final, summative evaluation at the semester's end. The debriefing experience, particularly during the semester as formative evaluation, is an excellent opportunity for students to apply learned content, think through rationales on which to base their actions, and clarify questions. It also enables students to evaluate their own critical thinking skills by comparing their rationale to that of other students and faculty.

Clinical Competencies

Clinical evaluation is multifaceted and often includes summative evaluation related to competencies. Technology is particularly useful in evaluating competencies with resources such as computer programs, learning labs, and HFPS. Further discussion of clinical evaluation with technology is included in chapters on simulation and clinical learning.

Emerging technologies provide clinical experiences in a safe and controlled environment, in which faculty can direct and control students' experiences. They also represent a fairly flexible teaching format that provides access to multiple students at their own convenience. Because of these features, technology provides a mechanism by which to address the Institute of Medicine's (IOM) goals. For example, the report on health professions education (IOM, 2003) calls for an emphasis on interdisciplinary education, but that is hard to accomplish when medical schools, nursing schools, and pharmacy schools all operate on very different schedules (for both didactic and clinical experiences). But a virtual hospital created in Second Life can provide the mechanism by which all three professions can work together, asynchronously if needed, so that incompatible schedules don't preclude the opportunity to work, learn, and practice concepts of interdisciplinary teamwork together. Potential for competency evaluation also exists via these venues.

TRIANGLE OF INTEGRATED LEARNING

The concept of integrated or deep learning achievement with technologies is central to this text. The content presented in this chapter falls soundly in the Integrated Learning Triangle; a major component in that triangle includes assessment, feedback, and evaluation. Fink (2003) describes these concepts as tools for learning. As discussed, technology provides many opportunities to help students achieve this integrated learning.

As discussed previously in the chapter, the evidence-based review abstract "Reflective Journaling" is provided in Exhibit 9.2. This synthesis of best evidence provides further direction for our work as educators.

SUMMARY

Technology provides faculty a wide variety of choices for providing student assessment, evaluation, and feedback. Optimizing various opportunities for feedback via assignment design creates multiple learning opportunities. Technologies such as online learning management systems create effective and efficient mechanisms for faculty use as well as student learning

Exhibit 9.2

EVIDENCE-BASED REVIEW ABSTRACT: REFLECTIVE JOURNALING

Compiled by: Janet Reagor, RN, MS

The Challenge

Reflective writing is useful in developing critical thinking skills, assisting in coping with stressful situations, and facilitating personal and professional growth. For reflective writing to be effective, the technique must be valued by the individual. Reflective writing is a skill that is developed with practice. By encouraging students to learn and develop reflective writing skills, they will hopefully continue to use this strategy after graduation where it may have an impact on their own growth and satisfaction in the role of the professional nurse, and have a positive impact on patient outcomes.

Synthesis/Interpretation of Current Literature

Journals are a widely accepted method to encourage students to reflect on both their successes and less than perfect performances during their clinical experiences. Journals encourage students to look beyond the facts of the incident, to explore the implications of the event, how alternative actions would have affected the event, and their own reactions to the event.

A systematic review of the literature supports use of reflection in clinical journals with opinions varying as to the role of grading journal entries. Many authors felt that grading the journal entries forced students to write not for their own benefit but to please the instructor. While some authors recommended the use of guided questions to facilitate student writing, other authors felt that this would stifle student creativity. All authors recommended that if journals are graded, they should be evaluated only on use of the reflective process, and not on the activities associated with the recorded incident. Several rubrics for evaluating the reflective process are available, varying widely in length, depth, and descriptors.

Ongoing Issues for Study

Several grading rubrics were found in the literature, but most were quite lengthy and would be time consuming for clinical instructors to use for grading. The ideal grading rubric should be short and clearly outline the process to be followed when writing the clinical journal. If, as many authors advocated, the journals are not graded, then further study on how to encourage students to be involved in the process of reflective journaling is needed.

Bibliography

Bilinski, H. (2002). The mentored journal. *Nurse Educator, 27,* 37–41.
Burton, A. J. (2000). Reflection: Nursing's practice and education panacea? *Journal of Advanced Nursing, 31,* 1009–1017.

(Continued)

Exhibit 9.2

EVIDENCE-BASED REVIEW ABSTRACT: REFLECTIVE JOURNALING (*Continued*)

Carroll, M., Curtis, L., Higgins, A., Nicholl, H., Redmond, R., & Timmins, F. (2002). Is there a place for reflective practice in the nursing curriculum? *Nurse Education in Practice, 2,* 13–20.

Craft, M. (2005). Reflective writing and nursing education. *Journal of Nursing Education, 44,* 53–57.

Duke, S., & Appleton, J. (2000). The use of reflection in a palliative care programme: A quantitative study of the development of reflective skills over an academic year. *Journal of Advanced Nursing, 32,* 1557–1568.

Epp, S. (2008). The value of reflective journaling in undergraduate nursing education: A literature review. *International Journal of Nursing Studies, 45,* 1379–1388.

Fonteyn, M. E., & Cahill, M. (1999). The use of clinical logs to improve nursing students' metacognition: A pilot study. *Journal of Advanced Nursing, 28,* 149–154.

Holmes, V. (1997). Grading journals in critical practice: A delicate issue. *Journal of Nursing Education, 36,* 489–491.

Ibarreta, G. I., & McLeod, L. (2004). Thinking aloud on paper: An experience in journal writing. *Journal of Nursing Education, 43,* 134–137.

Jensen, S. K., & Joy, C. (2005). Exploring a model to evaluate levels of reflection in baccalaureate nursing students' journals. *Journal of Nursing Education, 44,* 139–142.

Kennison, M. M. (2002). Evaluating reflective writing for appropriateness, fairness, and consistency. *Nursing Education Perspectives, 23,* 238–242.

Letcher, D. C., & Yancey, N. R. (2004). Witnessing change with aspiring nurses: A human becoming teaching-learning process in nursing education. *Nursing Science Quarterly, 17,* 36–41.

Plack, M. M., Driscoll, M., Blissett, S., McKenna, R., & Plack, T. P. (2005). A method for assessing reflective journal writing. *Journal of Allied Health, 34,* 199.

Riely-Doucet, C., & Wilson, S. (1997). A three-step method of self-reflection using reflective journal writing. *Journal of Advanced Nursing, 25,* 964–968.

Ruland, J. P., & Ahem, N. R. (2007). Transforming student perspectives through reflective writing. *Nurse Educator, 32,* 81–88.

opportunities. Human simulators are another example of technology as a tool for evaluating students' competencies and providing feedback. Technology provides both formative and summative evaluation opportunities to help guide student learning and progress toward independent clinical practice, interdisciplinary team work, and lifelong learning.

ENDING REFLECTION

1. What is the most important content that you learned in this chapter?
2. What are your plans for using the information in this chapter in your future teaching endeavors?
3. What are your further learning goals?

GUIDELINES FOR FEEDBACK, DEBRIEFING, AND EVALUATION WITH TECHNOLOGY

Quick Tips

1. Beginning assessments—whether at the beginning of a semester or the start of an individual class day—let both you and students know what knowledge gaps exist and identify what needs to be learned.
2. Use multiple sources for evaluation, and check between the sources for consistency (if consistency is lacking, consider possible explanations and their implications for student learning).
3. Always find something positive to say about student performance.

Questions for Further Reflection

1. Can all feedback be considered good feedback? What are some considerations related to this question?
2. What strategies do you currently use to provide formative feedback to students?
3. What strategies do you use to challenge students to self-reflect and set further learning goals? How do these strategies contribute to active learning and critical thinking?
4. What are the benefits and limitations of various technological options for evaluation?
5. Will the use of technological options such as simulation and gaming improve student learning in a meaningful way?
6. What information will you use to make a decision (in the Triangle of Integrated Learning) regarding which technology to use?
7. What do we mean by high- and low-stakes evaluation? What tools are used by other fields to measure and improve individual competency? Can those tools be applied to nursing?

8. What are benefits of competency-based education and training for individuals, for agencies, and for society?

Learning Activity

You are teaching a course in which students are presenting group projects on a semester-long community teaching activity. Your syllabus says the presentation evaluation will consist of self-evaluation, peer evaluation, and faculty evaluation.

1. What type of evaluation criteria or rubric will you expect each of these three rating groups to use?
2. If using a rubric, will each rating group (self, peer, and faculty) use the same rubric criteria? Whether you chose the same or different rubric criteria for each group, explain your rationale.

A year later you are teaching the same course. In trying to improve students' grades this year, you decide to add a formative project evaluation at mid-semester so that students get feedback as they work on the projects/presentations.

1. Will criteria you use for the mid-semester evaluation be the same or different from the evaluation criteria you use at the end of the semester? Explain the rationale for your decision.

Online Resources for Further Learning

- Carnegie Mellon, Teaching with Clickers. This site holds links to a variety of topics, including assessment and clickers: http://www.cmu.edu/teaching/index.html
- University of Virginia, Teaching Resource Center. This site contains links to numerous teaching resources, including "course evaluations" and "grading": http://trc.virginia.edu/Publications/Teaching_Concerns/TC_Topic.htm
- University of Wisconsin–Madison, National Institute for Science Education, Field-tests Learning Assessment Guide (FLAG). This site offers a variety of resources, including Classroom Assessment Techniques (CATs), through which you can find links to concept mapping and rubrics, among others: http://www.flaguide.org/

- Indiana University Kokomo, Center for Teaching, Learning, and Assessment. This site offers tips on assessment, including best practices for student assessment: http://www.iuk.edu/~koctla/assessment/9 principles.shtml

REFERENCES

American Association of Higher Education Assessment Forum. (1993). *Nine principles of good practice for assessing student learning.* Retrieved September 12, 2009, from http://www.aahe.org/assessment/principl.htm

Bastable, S. B. (2008). *Nurse as educator: Principles of teaching and learning for nursing practice.* Sudbury, MA: Jones and Bartlett.

Billings, D. M., & Halstead, J. A. (2009). *Teaching in nursing: A guide for faculty.* St. Louis, MO: Saunders Elsevier.

Bonnel, W., Ludwig, C., & Smith, J. (2007). Providing feedback in online courses: What do students want? How do we do that? *Annual Review of Nursing Education, 6,* 205–221.

Driscoll, A., & Wood, S. (2007). *Developing outcomes-based assessment for learner-centered education: A faculty introduction.* Sterling, VA: Stylus.

Fink, L. D. (2003). *Creating significant learning experiences: An integrated approach to designing college courses.* San Francisco: Jossey-Bass.

Institute of Medicine (IOM). (2003). *Health professions education: A bridge to quality.* Washington, DC: National Academies Press.

Shea, V. (1994). *Netiquette.* San Francisco: Albion Books.

Stevens, D., & Levi, A. (2005). *Introduction to rubrics.* Sterling VA: Stylus Publishing.

Tierney, R., & Simon, M. (2004). What's still wrong with rubrics: Focusing on the consistency of performance criteria across scale levels. *Practical Assessment, Research & Evaluation, 9*(2). Retrieved October 16, 2009, from http://pareonline.net/getvn.asp?v=9&n=2

Walvoord, B., & Anderson, V. (1998). *Effective grading: A tool for learning and assessment.* San Francisco: Jossey-Bass.

Diverse Clinical Practice and Educational Technologies

10 Online Education and Diverse Teaching and Learning Opportunities

CHAPTER GOAL

Consider best practices for teaching and learning in an online environment.

BEGINNING REFLECTION

1. What does the concept of online learning mean to you?
2. What are your best experiences teaching in an online environment? Your most challenging?

INTRODUCTION

Online learning has changed education by connecting diverse learners from around the globe. Online learning provides the opportunity to bring the world in, connecting beyond the confines of the learning management system. The Web makes it possible to connect with experts or resources from across the state or around the world.

Faculty have a baseline in traditional teaching modes, but are now facilitating learning in new ways online. Online learning has provided opportunities to reflect on our traditional teaching modes and examine what works and what does not in the online setting. Much has been written about the online classroom, as it has led to major changes in all arenas, including nursing education. Online education has presented a major stimulus for reconsidering our pedagogy as health care educators.

Both benefits and challenges exist in online education. While online education's benefits include flexibility for students, challenges often exist in engaging learners and making content interactive. Online learning is quite different from the classroom setting. Trying to create online the same effect as in a face-to-face classroom typically does not work. For example, just because it is now possible to lecture online does not necessarily mean that particular mode best accomplishes course objectives. This chapter focuses on online courses that meet entirely online without a face-to-face classroom component. An overview of opportunities and strategies for enhancing online courses for health professions students is provided. This chapter focuses on the pedagogy of online learning rather than the learning management systems.

WHY WE MEET OUR STUDENTS ONLINE

Learning online provides students advantages in a number of ways. Benefits of access and timeliness to online learning are key, including the ongoing access to course and Web resources, geographic flexibility, and time flexibility. The Web affords a wide variety of learning opportunities that help meet students' diverse learning styles and personal needs. Faculty actually have more opportunities for interaction with students, compared to scheduled weekly class sessions often held in the classroom. Faculty gain opportunities to receive comments from all students. Often students gain the opportunity to learn from diverse populations and gain access to a wide range of individuals that likely would not happen in one classroom.

Online and self-directed learning are particularly intertwined; online methods promote learner responsibility and preparation for self-directed learning. Fink (2003) points out that learning how to learn is a critical concept. In particular, online learning starts best with good orientations, not only to the course but also to learning online. Faculty guide or coach students in learning skills and concepts to prepare for the profession. Students gain opportunities in a structured venue for developing self-directed learning skills.

WHAT WE MEAN BY AN ONLINE COURSE

Terms for online education vary, incorporating terms such as "Web-based learning," "e-learning," "online learning," "virtual classes," and others. Palloff and Pratt (2001) note that trying to describe online education, with its rapidity of change, is like trying to describe a fast-moving river. Broad principles can provide direction in dealing with this rapidly evolving resource.

Online learning descriptions are also complicated by the additional concepts of synchronous and asynchronous learning. Synchronous learning describes experiences completed in real time. Asynchronous learning, such as used with online discussion boards, takes place at staggered times. Advantages to synchronous learning include real-time student interactions and feedback. Disadvantages include things such as time and place logistics with diverse students (Daniels & Pethel, 2005).

Online education, starting primarily as text-based learning, has grown rapidly to encompass a variety of teaching/learning opportunities and approaches. While online education has been offered with a book and study questions, much is missing if online courses are not expanded to incorporate educational best practices (see the following discussion of best practices). A major benefit to online education is the broad connections with the world; this link is missed if students are provided just a book and a study guide within the confines of a learning management system. Technology allows online courses to use a variety of features, including interactive assignments such as surveys, discussions, and authentic learning assignments (for example online student posters and presentations). Opportunities for applied assignments such as interviews and observations related to clinical learning are also available. These tools take us a long way in expanding on previously text-based online learning.

Particularly in online courses, engaging students to actively do something with the information presented is central in learning (Chickering & Ehrmann, 1996). For example, in an online nursing informatics class, reading a book and taking quizzes on content can be one approach. Using that approach, though, students lose many learning opportunities if they don't additionally engage in applied assignments and online discussions within the learning community. The latter approach helps students to further consider how the information applies in their own or future clinical settings.

BEST PRACTICES IN ONLINE TEACHING, SELECTED MODELS

What is the pedagogy behind the technology for online education? Best educational practices consistent with adult education theory are considered guides. Best classroom educational practices have been evaluated by Chickering and Ehrmann (1996) as having potential for best practices in online education as well. Evidence-supported learning practices described by Carnegie Mellon University (2009) are consistent with active learning. Based on best practices, optimal learning is more likely to occur if faculty do more than just choose a textbook and place a study guide online. Interactive courses help engage students in learning content. Examples of Web sites that support best practices in online education are listed in Exhibit 10.1.

Using best practices in teaching and learning as guides, the following concepts are discussed as tools for promoting successful online education: concepts of course design, facilitating applied active learning, and feedback to students.

Exhibit 10.1

WEB SITES THAT SUPPORT BEST PRACTICES

Web sites that support best practices in teaching/learning online education include:

- The Teaching, Learning, and Technology Group (TLT). This group provides faculty support in using changing technologies: http://www.tltgroup.org/
- Implementing the Seven Principles: Technology as Lever. This resource provides Chickering and Ehrmann's adaptation of classroom best practice for technologies in the online setting: http://www.Tltgroup.Org/Programs/Seven.Html
- Quality Matters. This organization provides resources and a systematic approach to quality review of online courses: http://www.qualitymatters.org/

CONCEPTS OF DESIGN IN ONLINE COURSES

Design and lesson planning concepts intertwine. Weimer (2002) described faculty as designers who create challenging assignments and then provide students the environment for success. Lesson plan principles guide the design phase as we move from classroom to online venues (our classroom teaching/learning experiences help us think about what we want to accomplish). Guided by the Integrated Learning Triangle (Appendix B) we use approaches similar to lesson plans but typically organize materials into a modular type electronic format. As discussed in Chapter 4, clear and relevant goals are critical to online assignment and course design.

As we move courses online, or design new courses in an online format, thinking about what needs to be retained from the classroom and what new strategies are needed provides direction for online design. Class organizing plans come in many shapes and sizes, and in almost all cases they influence classroom accomplishments. Similar in arrangement to more traditional learning modules, good formats include objectives, learning resources, and learning activities. Walvoord and Anderson (1998) cite the importance of integrating and aligning assessment (and feedback) with course learning goals and teaching/learning activities. They note that appropriate course design can help alleviate later problems in the course. As noted in the Integrated Learning Triangle (Appendix B), learning objectives, learning activities, and feedback and evaluation make up the points of the triangle, providing direction for course design as well.

Focusing on the assignments and relevant feedback that lead to course outcomes guides students in mastering content. One approach is to consider the big picture of the online course around course phases. Focusing on course phases (calendar view of the course) during the design phase maintains the teaching/learning flow from beginning to end (see Exhibit 10.2). These concepts provide direction for integrating technology and facilitating student learning in creating assignments that begin the course, move it along, and then bring closure.

When using best practices to facilitate learning with a "calendar" view of the course, "beginnings" acknowledge that learning communities are groups of people coming together with common learning goals. Strategies such as those noted in Exhibit 10.2 help diverse generations learn together with and about technologies. Addressing course "middles" recognizes the need for ongoing interesting activities to motivate learners. As faculty consider applications and authentic learning that can be a part

Exhibit 10.2

ONLINE TEACHING STRATEGIES TO BUILD THE LEARNING COMMUNITY

Designing courses that develop a robust online learning community can include a big picture calendar approach to a course. Attending to beginnings, middles, and endings in online course design promotes efficient course facilitation. Sample approaches to using concepts of beginnings, middles, and ending for organizing include the following:

Beginnings, Using Best Practices to Set the Stage for Learning

- Gain knowledge of the learners
- Orient learners to the class and to the technologies
- Create beginning class set

Middles/Transitions, Technologies and Facilitating Applied/Authentic Learning

- Make learning active and authentic to engage the learning community
- Create meaningful assignments
- Use our educator repositories (examples include Robert Wood Johnson Quality & Safety Education for Nurses resources)

Endings, Technologies, Feedback and Debriefing

- Use feedback and debriefing
- Use rubrics to promote feedback ease and reliability
- Assign students self-reflection activities and portfolios as opportunities to synthesize authentic learning
- Create class closure

of online learning, we have opportunities to expand students' views of the world. Specific to course endings, faculty have a coaching role in providing student feedback as well as debriefing intense learning experiences. Feedback and debriefing are especially important in online environments, helping deepen and cement student learning.

A variety of approaches help students learn online. Varying types of assignments allow diverse opportunities for interactions with content and help meet diverse learners' needs. Varied approaches such as voice, video, and print can be combined to create unique online learning opportunities. Questions can guide course decisions, such as: Do audio or video components enhance or support learning opportunities? What are the advantages and disadvantages of each in helping students learn and use information? Further questions to stimulate thinking about features to be designed into courses include the following. Will you:

- Incorporate audio or lecture online such as a podcast or classroom capture?
- Incorporate visuals (online videos/other)?
- Use applied assignments with interaction? (See further discussion below)
- Use group assignments?
- Use quizzes and responses to cases to provide a way to document attainment/mastery of the content?

O'Neil (2008) describes the benefits of a decision tree for making decisions about online course development. She additionally recommends a quality check of course pages as well as field testing and piloting online course modules prior to course start date. Copyright issues when using materials developed by others should also be considered.

FACILITATING APPLIED ACTIVE LEARNING

Applied learning assignments are particularly relevant to enhance interaction with content in online learning. While online education in the past was often text based, readings or written content presentations alone provide limited support of learning. Active learning involves working with the content in some way, such as applying it to cases or interacting via quizzes or other assignments. Engaging, active learning assignments help students use and understand the content.

Synthesis of research supports that active learning helps students gain and retain learning (Chickering & Gamson, 1986; Institute of Medicine, 2003). As with teaching in other settings, when students use active learning opportunities online to engage with a topic, content is better attended to. A variety of tools (for example cases, Web site reviews, and authentic assignments) paired with learning concepts can promote the integration of information needed to guide students in providing clinical care.

Cases

Case examples and problem-based learning provide an opportunity to visualize and bring to life concepts and processes. Cases involve learner–content interaction that requires critical thinking. The questioning that students bring to case study work and to problem-based learning helps them actively use concepts in preparing for clinical care. The questioning afforded by these methods helps them better put content into context, leading to enhanced clinical judgment and safety in care approaches (Benner, Tanner, & Chesla, 2009). Case study and other inquiry-based methods help students take responsibility for their learning as they identify issues, frame questions, seek resources, and identify care solutions (McKeachie & Svinicki, 2006) for their specialized clinical areas.

Web Site Reviews

While faculty have always focused on helping students with acquiring information, information is now so readily available that not only access but also critique is important. Weimer (2002) noted the need to discover how best to teach with a world at our fingertips. Benefits exist to extending courses beyond the confines of the learning management system to capture aspects of the broader world. Helping students use best-evidence Web resources, as discussed in Chapter 5, also serves as a tool for promoting self-directed and lifelong learning; students graduating as self-directed learners gain further learning opportunities from familiarity with important clinical web resources.

Authentic Assignments

Broad categories of interactive assignments include interview, observation, and document review (Bonnel & Meek, 2007). Discussed in Chapter 8, these tools provide flexibility in teaching to different types of learners and diverse groups. They also provide numerous opportunities for students to learn from each other's experiences. Sample ways students can explore and learn about clinical practice include the following:

- ***Developing applied products.*** Vella (2002) describes the importance of accountable learning online. Applied projects can include a project developed by students to demonstrate their learning while meeting a particular patient or population need in a clinical setting. Incorporating projects into learning plans builds on good educational practices and provides an authentic product for peer and faculty review.
- ***Interviews.*** Online sharing of interview summaries from mentors or others provides an opportunity to compare experiences and their similarities and differences in how things are done. For students,

interviews may even serve as access to new settings, providing introductions even to future mentors.

■ *Document reviews.* Sharing document reviews, such as patient education resources on the Web, students not only select an issue or problem to share but also review multiple teaching resources on the topic and consider the benefits or problems with each, selecting one as a tool for practice. As students share their work via online discussion groups, all students gain a variety of resources for their own practice.

■ *Observations.* Projects specific to "observation" type assignments such as patient education groups or support groups, in relevant courses, provide students an opportunity to learn about nursing care in a variety of settings. As students share summaries online of their experiences, the learning community often benefits from gaining diverse perspectives.

An example of authentic learning in a patient education nursing elective includes an observational assignment as noted above. In this observation assignment, students observe a group education session and complete a brief report. Students are then asked to share key bullets specific to the people, the place, and the process involved in the group education they observed. As students reflect and share in the online discussion, they gain information from these observations of educational groups in different settings (such as rural and urban), different clinical specialties, and different populations. Instead of learning teaching tips from only one group observation, a class of 20 students gains group teaching tips from 20 different educators. Further description of this course and teaching/learning examples are provided in Exhibit 10.3, with examples from a nursing elective in patient education.

Adding Reflection to Applied Learning

Adding reflection to applied learning further cements learning (Fink, 2003). For example, with applied learning projects, students can enhance their learning by reflecting and conversing with others about these experiences. Since students often complete applied learning projects at sites distant from each other, there are benefits to moving their reflections and discussions about these experiences online. Reflection promotes learning as students synthesize what they have learned and share their learning with others.

Exhibit 10.3

BSN ELECTIVE PATIENT EDUCATION FOR DIVERSE POPULATIONS, EXAMPLES OF APPLIED LEARNING

The patient education course for nurses completing their bachelor's degree provides opportunities for students to reflect on possible future educator roles. The course is designed to develop the health professional's role as patient educator and to promote a skill set to enhance teaching and learning for diverse multicultural patient populations. Students gain experiences assessing the learning needs of a target population and developing educational programs. Participants apply current learning theories and effective teaching strategies to design, implement, and evaluate educational experiences for diverse learners. Technological advances, as well as current and future issues in patient and clinical education, are considered.

Context

RN to BSN population. Active online participation has particular appeal for younger groups who see the Internet as a comfortable place to extend their learning.

Course Methods

Based on adult learning theory, the eight-module course integrates active learning and applied assignments. Online texts such as Healthy People 2010 and recent IOM reports on patient safety provide students easily accessible readings to complement more traditional resources.

Engaging Assignments

Students share cultural competence briefings with classmates; gain awareness of health literacy issues and communication tools; assess their practice sites for cultural competence; reflect on patient Web use and critique Web sites for their educational potential; gain a skill set for actively involving patients in their learning; identify new evaluation approaches; and critique interdisciplinary patient education approaches. An applied project in the form of a teaching plan that students pilot in patient care is included as well.

Process

Assignments are designed with an applied focus including interviews of an experienced patient educator, observations of a patient education group teaching session, and reviews of online patient teaching resources. The majority of students' assignments are then shared in summary format at an online discussion board.

Additionally students review online resources to enhance student cultural competence and patient teaching for diverse populations. A sample assignment is a cultural debriefing provided to student colleagues at an online discussion board. Health promotion Web sites with topic relevance for a patient health promotion teaching session such as Healthy People 2010 are used.

(*Continued*)

Exhibit 10.3

BSN ELECTIVE PATIENT EDUCATION FOR DIVERSE POPULATIONS, EXAMPLES OF APPLIED LEARNING (*Continued*)

Benefits and Evaluation

Access to diverse Web sites and applied learning experiences provides students authentic learning that transfers to their future practice. Web sites reviewed are available for students to catalog for future clinical practice. Using the active learning strategies gives students practice in becoming more self-directed learners.

Student fast feedback forms, student projects, course evaluations and student surveys from this RN to BSN elective support that students like the approach, learn educator skills, and in many cases expand their thinking to consider future faculty roles.

Discussion Groups Online

Online discussions often serve as a central focus of an online course, serving as a way for the online learning community to connect and share. Text-based discussions (missing classroom immediacy as well as verbal and nonverbal prompts) change the context for faculty and student discussions and questioning. Technology brings online discussion opportunities that allow unique ways of bringing diverse groups together. Some tips for interesting, successful discussions include the following:

- Clearly identify faculty roles (and expectations) as well as student roles in participating and processing discussions.
- Provide orientation and clear guidelines as to the discussion purpose and process.
- Provide interesting topics such as those with controversy, including interesting discussion prompts as the discussion progresses.
- Consider strategies for facilitating evaluation of discussions, including the use of rubrics that help guide discussion purposes and outcomes.
- Synthesize course discussions to summarize, reinforce, and give meaning to patterns emerging in online course discussions.

As part of online discussions, questions serve as a way to engage students. Brookfield and Preskill (2005) discussed teaching as a blend of conversations and questioning, noting the culture of inquiry promoted by questions. While many questioning techniques utilized in the traditional classroom can be transferred to the online classroom, qualities such as wait time, eye contact, and tone are not available in text-based courses.

Online education presents a unique opportunity for enhancing the use of questions. Faculty can get a snapshot of students' thinking processes via questioning. Purposeful questions add an active component via approaches such as:

- Guiding student reflections on a particular topic. When questions are in the form of a student survey, for example, faculty can generate reports and then provide group feedback on the results or generate further questions for discussion.
- Summarizing responses to a clinical experience. Questions guide student reflections after clinical activities. For example, at the end of the clinical week in a clinical course students complete and send a summary and e-mail responding to the following questions: What's the best thing that happened? What was the most challenging thing?
- Guiding students with questions that help them reflect on what they are learning within specific modules adds an active learning component even to readings. Asking students to consider and share the three most important or interesting points for their practice from a reading supports learning of the community as well.

FEEDBACK TO STUDENTS ONLINE

Feedback in online education provides students information on their achievements. Faculty-friendly ways exist to provide feedback in this unique learning medium. Whether feedback is part of a discussion, a sequenced progressive project, or brief assignment activities, it is a way to support learning and to promote student connection with the learning community. Appropriate feedback helps students gauge their learning progress and take further responsibility for their learning (Bonnel, 2008). Chapter 9 provides further information about feedback as a broad concept.

All online assignments are not created equal for feedback. Designing assignments with fit for good feedback and linking these assignments to course objectives are consistent with the Integrated Learning Triangle (Appendix B). Assignment design includes considering if different types of feedback are needed at different points in the semester (perhaps related to maintaining course momentum and student learning). Other considerations include the following:

- Build student skills in seeking feedback, giving students permission to request additional feedback and guiding the best and most timely ways to access faculty.
- Designate selected assignments for the most focused feedback. For example, clarify with students that different types of assignments such as "Learning Activities" are for their own reflection and do not require extensive faculty feedback.
- Use templates for more efficiency in feedback. Automated grade books provide opportunities for timesaving templates that can be individualized with a phrase or two.
- Enhance opportunities for self-assessment, a type of self-feedback.
- Train students in use of rubrics to provide peer feedback on selected assignments.

Additional feedback issues in the course design phase include the pacing of the course assignments. Faculty will want to consider assignment depth, breadth, and the time frame for completion of assignments and feedback. Major projects that build across the semester provide opportunities for multiple feedback opportunities before the product is finished. A faculty survey (Bonnel & Boehm, 2008) found that three broad categories of approaches guided faculty in efficient and effective ways to provide feedback:

- Having a system for feedback. Examples included being proactive and minimizing potential student problems through early guidance and restating/clarifying expectations.
- Using best available tools. Examples included using rubrics, templates, and automated responses to assessing knowledge and increasing efficiency of feedback response.
- Creating feedback-rich environments. Examples included use of assignments such as journal writing or self-assessment to stimulate students' self-examination and introspection in order to evaluate performance and stimulate critical thinking skills.

An evidence-based review abstract, "Seeking Best Evidence, Promoting Online Integrity," is shared at chapter end. This systematic review provides faculty direction for promoting online integrity. Strategies for proactively focusing on honesty in the online setting can help students focus on the positive ethical approaches to learning online.

CONTINUOUS QUALITY IMPROVEMENT AND ONLINE EDUCATION

As reflective educators, we take opportunities to look back at courses and assignments and determine what has been helpful and what has not in helping students learn. We gain opportunities to revise or reshape those course components that are least successful. Consistent with the "Revise" component of the Integrated Learning Triangle (Appendix B), continuous quality improvement (CQI) in a course builds on this faculty reflection. For example, the authors' evaluation practice typically includes seeking ongoing course module evaluations and student final semester evaluations in conjunction with student activities throughout the semester (course project quality and student grades, for example). Then, after reflecting on this information, relevant themes are noted and appropriate changes made to the course structure or process. Faculty course reflections can often lead to piloting new teaching and learning strategies.

Ongoing module evaluations can provide rapid input from students as to what works in a course assignment or what does not. A useful tool to gain quick student feedback on modules or assignments is asking students to complete fast feedback forms with modules, answering the following questions:

- What worked?
- What did not?
- What would you like to see changed?

Tools such as those developed by the Teaching, Learning, and Technology Group (2004) provide students with more formal opportunities to look back and rate the usefulness of an online course or assignment. Among other programs, the Quality Matters program is a faculty-centered, peer-review process designed to certify the quality of online courses and online components. The Quality Matters rubric consists of eight broad standards that identify desired outcomes and clarify acceptable evidence to show these are met, including the following (Quality Matters, 2006)

1. Course Overview and Introduction
2. Learning Objectives
3. Assessment and Measurement
4. Resources and Materials
5. Learner Engagement
6. Course Technology

7. Learner Support
8. Accessibility

Further discussion is needed across nursing education that focuses on teaching best practices, evaluation, and CQI with online education; there is also a need to generate further research questions related to best practices.

USING LEARNING MANAGEMENT SYSTEMS FOR ONLINE EDUCATION

Pedagogy and new technologies promote new ways of teaching/learning with learning management systems as a major part of online learning. Discussed in Chapter 9, these technologies include features that can mimic the classroom. Features commonly useful in learning management systems include the following online options:

- Distribute course materials
- Post grades for students to access
- Provide student surveys with online results tracking
- Interact with class participants via discussion boards or chat features
- Create and administer tests or integrate with test software

A focus on the learning as well as the management functions in learning management systems provides enhanced teaching and learning opportunities. Particularly with online learning, we want students to spend most of their time learning the content and not learning the technology. Facilitating optimal learning time includes focus on the following:

- Orienting students to the learning management system; ideally a technology support person will be available to students.
- Helping students be clear on what learning will be like online. Addressing not only the learning management system but the process for learning in the course, this orientation can highlight the roles of faculty and students, the types and purposes of varied assignments, and their work as guided learners with self-directed emphasis. This might be in the form of letters to students about the course and documents with student guidelines.

As discussed previously in the chapter, the evidence-based review abstract "Seeking Best Evidence, Promoting Online Integrity" is provided in Exhibit 10.4. This synthesis of best evidence provides further direction for our work as educators.

Exhibit 10.4

EVIDENCE-BASED REVIEW ABSTRACT: SEEKING BEST EVIDENCE, PROMOTING ONLINE INTEGRITY

Compiled by: Amanda L. Alonzo, PhD, RN

Challenge

As an increasing number of nursing programs are developing online and Web-enhanced formats, many faculty question the ability to ensure honesty and integrity in the online environment. Incorporating best practices in online honesty and integrity is essential to ensuring the rigor of nursing education. A systematic review of the literature identified best practices in promoting online student integrity.

Sample Best Practices

Based on best literature evidence, best practices for promoting student honesty and integrity include utilizing a log-in system, particularly for online assessments; frequent faculty–student communication through e-mail; discussion boards and chats to become familiar with individual students' writing style; incorporating a code of ethics in each course; using online software/Web sites to detect plagiarism in student work; and creating assignments to maximize student honesty and integrity.

Model Case

A workshop was presented to expose faculty to best practices in promoting honesty and integrity in online learning and to provide an opportunity to utilize these strategies in assignments. Following a presentation on preventing plagiarism in written work, faculty worked on sample individual assignments to identify plagiarism and then worked on creating a sequenced progressive assignment designed to minimize opportunities for plagiarism.

Implications

Potential implications for implementing best practices in online honesty and integrity include faculty awareness and utilization of best practices and faculty experience in use of best practice techniques.

Summary Recommendations

Implementation of best practices in online honesty and integrity is essential to ensure the quality of online nursing education. Through awareness of best literature evidence, nursing faculty will be better prepared to offer quality nursing education in an online course environment that promotes honesty and integrity.

(*Continued*)

Exhibit 10.4

EVIDENCE-BASED REVIEW ABSTRACT: SEEKING BEST EVIDENCE, PROMOTING ONLINE INTEGRITY (*Continued*)

Bibliography

Anna, D. J. (1998). Computerized testing in a nursing curriculum: A case study. *Nurse Educator, 23*(4), 22–26.

Carnevale, D. (2007). *Your cheatin' heart.* Retrieved May 24, 2007, from http://chronicle.com/wiredcampus/article/2086/your-cheatin-heart

Gaberson, K. B. (1997). Academic dishonesty among nursing students. *Nursing Forum, 32*(3), 14–21.

Gibbons, A., Mize, C. D., & Rogers, K. L. (2002). That's my story and I'm sticking to it: Promoting academic integrity in the online environment. *Association for the Advancement of Computing in Education.* Presented at the 2002 World Conference on Educational Multimedia, Hypermedia & Telecommunications, Denver, Colorado, June 24–29.

Kiernan, V. (2005). Show your hand, not your ID. *The Chronicle of Higher Education, 52*(15). Retrieved June 28, 2007, from http://chronicle.com/weekly/v52/i15/15a02801.htm

Koeckeritz, J., Malkiewicz, J., & Henderson, A. (2002). The seven principles of good practice: Applications for online education in nursing. *Nurse Educator, 27*(6), 283–287.

Heberling, M. (2002). Maintaining academic integrity in online education. *Online Journal of Distance Learning Administration, 5*(1). Retrieved June 28, 2007, from http://www.westga.edu/~distance/ojdla/spring51/heberling51.html

Langone, M. (2007). Promoting integrity among nursing students. *Journal of Nursing Education, 46*(1), 45–47.

Olt, M. (2002). Ethics and distance education: Strategies for minimizing academic dishonesty in online assessment. *Online Journal of Distance Learning Administration, 5*(3). Retrieved June 28, 2007, from http://www.westga.edu/~distance/ojdla/fall53/olt53.html

Palerma, J., & Evans, A. (2006). Relationships between personal values and reported behavior on ethical scenarios for law students. *Behavioral Sciences and the Law, 25*(1), 121–136.

Pevoto, B. (2000). *Advising challenges in cyberspace.* Presented at the Annual Conference of the Association for Career and Technical Education/International Vocational Education and Training Association.

Rubens, A. J., & Wimberley, E. T. (2004). Contrasting the American college of healthcare executives' code of ethics with undergraduate health administration students' values and ethical decision choices. *Hospital Topics, 82*(3), 10–17.

Scanlon, C. L. (2006). Strategies to promote a climate of academic integrity and minimize student cheating and plagiarism. *Journal of Allied Health, 35*(3), 179–185.

Shyles, L. (2002). *Authenticating, identifying, and monitoring learners in the virtual classroom: Academic integrity in distance learning.* Paper presented at the Annual Meeting of the National Communication Association.

SUMMARY

Online education provides amazing opportunities to engage students in learning course concepts and to create enhanced learning using a world of resources. Faculty teaching strategies based on best practices include the concepts of design, facilitation, and feedback. A focus on beginnings, middles, and endings of courses provides further direction in course facilitation. While face-to-face classroom learning and clinical experiences do not automatically come online, there are great opportunities for blending these approaches with online education.

ENDING REFLECTION

1. What is the most important content that you learned in this chapter?
2. What are your plans for using the information in this chapter in your future teaching endeavors?
3. What are your further learning goals?

GUIDELINES FOR ONLINE EDUCATION AND DIVERSE TEACHING AND LEARNING OPPORTUNITIES

Quick Tips for Teaching Online

1. Have a big picture of what should be accomplished in the course. Working backwards in designing courses from the point of outcomes desired provides useful perspective.
2. Consider how many ways students' real world experiences can be incorporated into online discussions.
3. Develop a learning community that provides students valued roles in self-assessment and peer review.

Questions for Further Reflection

1. Does being a good classroom teacher make you a good online teacher? What are similarities and differences?
2. What are essential principles of good practice in online teaching? What examples of these principles come to mind for you to draw on?

3. What are the best ways to assess and engage diverse learning styles in online courses?
4. How is feedback different in online courses from that in face-to-face classes? In what ways do student and faculty roles specific to feedback change in the online setting? How do we know students are using and benefiting from feedback?
5. What are examples of strategies you use to promote self-assessment, peer review, and group work for feedback?

Learning Activity: Designing Opportunities for Online Feedback

Considering a course you are currently teaching (or would like to teach), how many of the following ways do you (or could you) integrate feedback into your online class?

Sample questions for each strategy (based on type of course; level of students; and course objectives) include: how should I use the strategy, when should I use it, how much weight do I attach to it, and what is gained by this approach?

1. Self-Evaluation/Reflection
2. Groups Assignments for Feedback
3. Peer Critique Strategies
4. Feedback From Others (Mentors/Course Guests)
5. Automated Feedback With Rubrics
6. Feedback From Faculty

Online Resources for Further Learning

- Keys to Facilitating Online Discussions. A variety of tips and activities for enhancing discussions are shared from the University of Wisconsin–Eau Claire: http://www.uwsa.edu/ttt/raleigh.htm
- NLN Living Books Best Practices in Online Learning. A publication on best practices to promote successful online learning experiences: http://electronicvision.com/nln/chapter02/index.htm

REFERENCES

Benner, P., Tanner, C., & Chesla, C. (2009). *Expertise in nursing practice: Caring, clinical judgment, and ethics* (2nd ed.). New York: Springer Publishing.

Bonnel, W. (2008). Improving feedback to students in online courses. *Nursing Education Perspectives, 29*(5), 290–294.

Bonnel, W., & Boehm, H. (2008). *Faculty practices in providing online course feedback.* Midwest Nursing Research Society Conference, Indianapolis.

Bonnel, W., & Meek, V. (2007). Qualitative assignments to enhance online learning communities. *Instructional Technology and Distance Learning, 4*(2), 49–54.

Brookfield, S., & Preskill, S. (1999). *Discussion as a way of teaching: Tools and techniques for democratic classrooms.* San Francisco: Jossey-Bass.

Carnegie Mellon University. (2009). *Enhancing education: Learning principles.* Retrieved October 4, 2009, from http://www.cmu.edu/teaching/principles/

Chickering, A., & Ehrmann, S. (1996). *Implementing the seven principles: Technology as lever.* Retrieved October 4, 2009, from http://www.tltgroup.org/programs/seven.html

Chickering, A. W., & Gamson, Z. F. (1986). *Seven principles for good practice in undergraduate education.* Retrieved October 4, 2009, from http://honolulu.hawaii.edu/intranet/committees/FacDevCom/guidebk/teachtip/7princip.htm

Daniels, T., & Pethel, M. (2005). Computer mediated communications. In M. Orey (Ed.), *Emerging perspectives on learning, teaching, and technology.* Retrieved October 4, 2009, from http://projects.coe.uga.edu/epltt/

Fink, L. D. (2003). *Creating significant learning experiences: An integrated approach to designing college courses.* San Francisco: Jossey-Bass.

Institute of Medicine. (2003). *Health professions education: A bridge to quality.* Retrieved October 4, 2009, from http://www.nap.edu/catalog.php?record_id=10681

McKeachie, W., & Svinicki, M. (2006). Problem-based learning: Teaching with cases, simulations, and games. In W. McKeachie & M. Svinicki (Eds.), *McKeachie's teaching tips: Strategies, research, and theory for college and university teachers* (12th ed.). Boston, MA: Houghton Mifflin.

O'Neil, C. (2008). Reconceptualizing the online course. In C. O'Neil, C. Fisher, & S. Newbold (Eds.), *Developing online learning environments in nursing education.* New York: Springer Publishing.

Palloff, R., & Pratt, K. (2001). *Lessons from the cyberspace classroom.* San Francisco: Jossey-Bass.

Quality Matters. (2006). *The Quality Matters rubric.* Retrieved October 16, 2009, from http://www.qualitymatters.org/Rubric.htm

Teaching, Learning, and Technology Group. (2004). *Resources.* Retrieved January 10, 2010, from http://www.tltgroup.org/resources.htm

Vella, J. (2002). *Learning to listen, learning to teach: The power of dialogue in educating adults* (rev. ed.). San Francisco: Jossey-Bass.

Walvoord, B., & Anderson, V. (1998). *Effective grading: A tool for learning and assessment.* San Francisco: Jossey-Bass.

Weimer, M. (2002). *Learner-centered teaching: Five key changes to practice.* San Francisco: Jossey-Bass.

The Changing Classroom and Technology

CHAPTER GOAL

Gain strategies for using technology in the changing classroom to promote student learning for safety and quality in patient care.

BEGINNING REFLECTION

1. What have been your most positive recent experiences with the changing classroom and technologies? The most challenging experiences?
2. What goals do you have for further use of technologies in the changing classroom?

INTRODUCTiON

Changing student populations, more rapid proliferation of information, and more technology resources lead to use of the classroom in new ways. In the past, faculty may have had huge notebooks of information they verbally imparted to students. Now students access online PowerPoint presentations and create additional learning tips via combinations of the lecture and Web reviews. For some faculty, the changing classroom means using clickers or audience response systems; for others it means bringing real-time video of simulations to students in the classroom. Technology is changing our uses of the classroom including different approaches to space, time, and structure (Malloch, 2009).

In traditional classrooms, students were often positioned as passive learners or class participants. Research on how people learn supports the finding that people learn best by being actively engaged and that different tools or technologies work best for different tasks (Commission on Behavioral and Social Sciences and Education, 1999). As students change from being passive classroom learners, technologies bring many opportunities for extending active learning roles and outcomes. The question then becomes how to best use technologies in order to achieve an effective balance or blend of classroom support and challenges. Technology can also increase ties to clinical experiences by bringing clinical cases and observations into the classroom via the Internet and easily accessible videos.

Changing the classroom may present initial challenges related to the more traditional teaching models, in which students expected their teachers to take the stage and provide a lecture. Weimer (2002) describes the changing function of course content, describing content as an opportunity for learning engagement, suggesting that content be used in class rather than merely covered. This shift promotes students' self-awareness as learners, their understanding of how they learn, and their ability to learn more as they gain new skill sets. Benner, Tanner, and Chesla (2009) note, for example, that cases and questions help move classroom theory to patient care in the clinical setting. This chapter describes strategies for combining the best of the traditional teaching/learning strategies with new, rapidly changing technologies.

While faculty no longer need an actual classroom to provide a course or even a lecture, there are advantages to a physical classroom. Students bring diverse interests and reasons for being in the classroom. The classroom brings historical perspectives (the familiarity of the learning setting that most students grew up with). It also offers pedagogical opportunities that can be enhanced with technology. The classroom setting may be particularly important for beginning learners. In the classroom, faculty have the opportunity to personalize learning, convey enthusiasm, model critical thinking, and enliven text-based information (Bradshaw & Lowenstein, 2006). Additional classroom benefits include the following:

- There can be an intensity or intimacy of learning. Faculty and students have the advantage of face-to-face conversations and can gain the immediate feel of a community.
- Faculty have more opportunities for modeling professional behaviors. We can read the body language of students. Clarifications in communications or follow-up questions can immediately occur.

Faculty use the classroom in different ways at different times. Students come to classrooms with different knowledge and mental sets at different points in time. As we think about our pedagogies for helping students move from backgrounds of limited knowledge to skill sets for managing complex patient care, we may need to put additional focus on Benner's (2001) novice to expert transitions. Different teaching technologies may be needed to support students at different points in time in learning different student skill sets.

Technology allows us to easily bring active learning into the classroom by using strategies such as student self-assessments, applied case studies, quiz questions embedded in PowerPoint presentations, and projects with clinical applications. Examples of clinical applications are evidence-based posters or patient care materials that use the course content in authentic ways. This chapter provides an overview of interactive learning opportunities with technology in the classroom, the classroom as an opportunity for extending distance learning, and the role of learning management systems.

TOOLS FOR MAKING THE LECTURE INTERACTIVE

Automated Response Systems or Clickers in the Classroom

Automated response systems, sometimes referred to as clickers or as classroom response or audience response systems, bring new opportunities into the classroom to promote critical thinking. Whether using clickers for case studies, opinion polls, or quizzes, students are encouraged to actively participate in content review, creating opportunities for practice testing and knowledge sharing. These clickers or wireless devices (typically purchased by students at the bookstore prior to class) provide faculty with the opportunity to survey or question students and then receive responses as students click their answers via the hand-held response system. Bruff (2009) describes the benefits of these tools, including class-wide discussion, homework review, and peer teaching. He also notes the important teacher responsibility in framing effective questions to promote student learning. The benefits and structuring of follow-up discussions to avoid sharing answers too soon and providing opportunities for students to share their rationale are also described.

There are as many ways to use clickers as there are to frame different types of survey and quiz questions, varying from agree/disagree responses to multiple choice. Relevant to broad content and process topics, clickers give students the opportunity to review course material and to practice test taking in preparation for standardized exams. They also provide faculty snapshot assessments of students' knowledge. Literature has supported that these devices are motivational and beneficial in learning. An evidence-based review abstract on automated response systems is provided at chapter end. Finding the right balance of automated-response use may be an issue, with further research needed on this topic.

Active Learning and PowerPoint: Making the Lecture Interactive

Active learning and PowerPoint are a good mix when combined for interactive classroom presentation. An interactive PowerPoint presentation builds in reminders for interaction with students. Weimer (2002) describes the importance of actively using content for learning rather than for merely covering the content in class.

There has been debate about PowerPoint uses in the classroom, with some educators suggesting that the tool creates passive learners (Rocklin, 1999). In the past, PowerPoint presentations gained a reputation for being only bulleted lists of topical information that, while informative, were often difficult for students to retain. When coupled with active learning activities that engage the audience, bulleted information lists are better retained. Asking students, for example, to apply selected bullets to a brief case application provides enhanced learning opportunities. The interactive lecture not only organizes content, highlighting the must-know information, but also engages students in learning the information. PowerPoint strengths include the following:

- It meets the needs of diverse learners, providing opportunities to engage the learners' hearing and visual senses, engaging those with both auditory and visual learning preferences.

- It addresses needs of visual learners with the visual benefits of PowerPoint in terms of showing diagrams and concept relationships. There are good opportunities for visual cues and opportunity to focus on the visual benefits such as providing a wound picture for students to assess and then asking students to document their findings.
- It provides a structure for organizing learning concepts, helping faculty remain organized in classroom presentations. It provides learners with neat, legible notes, supporting both prior reading and in-class note taking.
- It serves as a strategy to engage the audience. Changing the pace of the presentation with an active learning approach can be a useful strategy to keep students engaged.

When using interactive lectures, with or without PowerPoint, or automated response systems, active learning opportunities can be provided. A good beginning question for faculty to consider is, "How am I using the technology, and is it to everyone's advantage?" Examples of various Power-Point strategies for engaging learners are included in Exhibit 11.1. In reviewing this information, note that all of these approaches are amenable to questions used with automated response systems or by students simply raising their hands in response to questions.

Exhibit 11.1

SAMPLE ACTIVE LEARNING OPPORTUNITIES FOR INTERACTIVE POWERPOINT PRESENTATIONS

Cases

Cases are a good way to illustrate points being made on an earlier slide. These cases promote retention as students apply the content to a case, since it is often easier to remember cases than a list of bulleted facts. Combining the two is a good strategy.

Stories

Stories of clinical practice help tie concepts/theory to practice. There is limited teaching value, for example, if content taught is not related to or modeled in clinical settings (Institute of Medicine, 2003). Determining best strategies for using technologies such as video, robotics, and telehealth to help students gain and transfer

(Continued)

Exhibit 11.1

SAMPLE ACTIVE LEARNING OPPORTUNITIES FOR INTERACTIVE POWERPOINT PRESENTATIONS (*Continued*)

information from classroom to clinical settings will provide ongoing questions for study.

Reflective Prompts and Discussion Questions

Active learning activities can include discussion opportunities during the Power-Point presentation. After covering broad key points on a topic, pertinent questions/prompts to promote reflection and use of the content can lead to further discussion. Key themes from the discussion can be noted on the white board. Students can incorporate the synthesized information into their notes.

Multiple Choice

Multiple-choice practice test questions can be used as a review for an upcoming exam. Students have an opportunity to learn from each other as the class discusses the correct answer and provides explanations for the incorrect responses.

Pair/Share Activities

General guides for this activity include providing a question, asking student pairs to discuss the question for 2 minutes, and then calling on selected groups to share summary points from their discussion.

Organizing Cues

Organized PowerPoint handouts are helpful in student learning, especially when used in conjunction with the required reading. In a pathophysiology course, for example, it would be appropriate to suggest that students review the PowerPoint handouts prior to class, making additional notes in the margins from information gathered from the readings.

Surveys/Debriefing

Stopping the class for an opinion poll on a specific question with potential for multiple perspectives promotes critical thinking and reflection.

WEB-BASED MODULES AS A CLASSROOM ADJUNCT

The Web can be used for education and teaching on almost any topic. Using the Internet to provide supplementary (or required) health care information can be a time-efficient approach for educators. This information is useful particularly as we seek to have students be prepared for classroom sessions and want to challenge them to use concepts after the class is completed (Fink, 2003). Products such as Web-based review modules provide benefit as a classroom adjunct.

Virtual tours are one example of an easy to develop assignment for classroom use based on Web resources (Bonnel, Fletcher, & Wingate, 2007). A virtual tour provides a package of educational materials based on Web resources that students can use to learn the materials now and to keep as a resource for future review. Used as tools to build on students' current knowledge levels, virtual tours can be quickly skimmed brief modules or more detailed modules for enhanced learning. For example, after a class on the care of patients with dementia, students may not recall all the unique facts of family caregiving with dementia patients, but they can likely recall a good Web-based resource for future use. Access to the Web site for support group resources and patient education information provides a useful ongoing clinical tool. As students continue to access the Alzheimer's Association Web site, they will also find the most current information including updates on treatments and research.

Virtual tours can be used as a type of homework or for pre- or postclass discussion preparation. Also, to extend independent learning, students can be asked to become familiar with the Web resources that provide information on specialty topics of interest. This might include, for example, parish nursing resources or evidence-based summaries from organizations such as those focused on palliative care.

TECHNOLOGY FOR MANAGING CLASSROOMS: LEARNING MANAGEMENT SYSTEMS

While this book is about pedagogies for teaching with technologies, it is worthwhile to also consider the management functions provided by technology in the classroom. Learning management systems are tools, such as Blackboard, that make it easier to organize our classes. They provide a variety of ways to manage classroom activities, including communication, distribution of course materials, and grading. Instead of copying volumes of information for students and carrying this to classrooms, we can now develop and organize our class documents in learning management systems. Students can print what they want and use electronic versions as they need, easily accessing class notes, class study guides, and other resources. Examples of options include the following:

- Organizing assignments or course grades
- Providing additional resources and Web sites for review

- Providing practice tests and online reviews
- Offering opportunities for student surveys
- Providing item analyses on tests
- Providing course calendars with assignment due dates
- Providing study and project guides

Basic communication features of learning management systems, such as announcement features, e-mail, and discussion boards, all promote enhanced communication with and between students and faculty. Drop box features, serving as collection resources for student assignments, enhance opportunities for providing feedback and making grades easily accessible to students. As we seek efficient, effective education, learning management systems provide tools to accomplish classroom management tasks.

While classroom management is enhanced with these tools, learning management systems also become tools that help faculty facilitate learning with good pedagogical principles. Assignments and project activities can be incorporated in new ways with tools such as discussion boards, blogs, and wikis for group sharing. Much more benefit can be achieved with these tools beyond being used as receptacles for delivering and receiving class materials. Sample strategies enhanced within the learning management system include:

- Organizing students into groups for project work or discussions. Learning management systems provide ways to extend assignment and classroom discussions, whether they are synchronous or asynchronous. In order to summarize readings, students might have discussion boards where they are assigned to share the three most interesting things they learned from readings.
- Gaining preclass assignments from which faculty can then select examples to share and build on during class (Bean, 1996). For example, question sets can be posted online prior to class for students to respond to. Answers and examples provided allow opportunity for faculty to share excerpts in class, bringing in personal student examples that quickly involve their diverse students. A similar approach can be used asking students to share case examples or experiences, such as previous work with particular patient populations.
- Additionally, technology can be used to guide students' informal writing to promote learning in larger classes, for example using slide prompts to encourage brief summary notes (or further questions to explore).

ALTERNATE CLASSROOM EXPERIENCE FOR STUDENTS AT A DISTANCE

Distance education has a long history and has even changed the ways that we think about classrooms. There are now tools available, such as classroom capture, online lecture, and interactive online voice-over PowerPoint for our work with distant students. These unique opportunities take representations of the classroom to the students. Distance education literature (Willis, 2004) has provided guidance in making classroom-type opportunities available to students at sites distant from the traditional classroom. In reviewing the following technologies that provide opportunities for distance education, it is useful to consider which of the traditional classroom strategies are most beneficial to retain in distance learning. For example, while lecture can be used in these formats as a teaching strategy, traditional lecture formats can create passive learners.

What are some of the approaches that attempt to provide a classroom setting at a distance when our students do not come to the traditional classroom? The classroom moves to multipoint conferencing software, such as Elluminate-type programs or Camtasia (merging tools for screen capture and audio-video recording to provide the classroom effect).

- **Web Conferencing Software.** Products such as Elluminate are considered Web conferencing software. These tools provide faculty real-time presentation opportunities with white boards, presentation software, and other tools. Students and faculty have the opportunity to communicate in real time verbally or in writing.
- **Classroom Capture Software.** If students do not come to class (for whatever reason), classroom capture software exists such as Camtasia that can provide much of the classroom experience as the student watches a video of the class.
- **Audio Casts.** Tools to create podcasts and voice-over PowerPoint presentations provide unidirectional audio broadcasts that promote opportunity for a more traditional lecture. Creative thinking with PowerPoint presentations (as noted above) provide faculty opportunities to promote an engaging climate with these presentations.
- **Interactive Television (ITV).** As faculty and students seek strategies to connect with others at a distance, teaching and learning are extended to multiple classrooms via interactive television (or the receiving and sending of audio and video via an Internet protocol address). Interactive television allows large, real-time classrooms at

distant sites to be engaged for interaction with faculty. Additionally, desktop or Web camera applications exist for a variety of conferencing systems for individual desktop conferencing and small conference rooms.

With any of the visual mediums, good pedagogy includes focus on positive use of both verbal and nonverbal cues in classroom presentations. Verbal cues include, for example, accepting and reacting to students' emotions, providing positive reinforcement, giving appropriate classroom feedback to students, and using questioning as a learning tool. Positive nonverbal cues such as eye contact, facial expressions, posture, and energy level help convey content as well as appropriate use of gestures, mannerisms, and movement in the classroom (Bailey, 1981).

Students using any of the previously noted distance learning resources might gain for example information for learning advanced practice nursing care. A statewide collaboration in Kansas, (C. Teel, personal communication, 2009), brings opportunities to share expertise from practitioners at universities across the state via a statewide repository of lectures and interactive learning materials. Students across the state learn in their homes from clinical experts across the state as these experts share voice-over PowerPoint presentations on varied topics, as well as provide interactive content quizzes and assignments.

Additional technologies can be used in connection with these tools to create learning communities that provide a more social feel of the classroom. For example, professional networking sites similar to social sites such as Facebook present potential for building professional peer involvement. Skiba (2008) describes the benefits of sharing professionally in a specialty area within these communities and describes low-cost options for doing this.

As discussed previously in the chapter, the evidence-based review abstract "Listening for a 'Click' in Classrooms" is provided in Exhibit 11.2. This synthesis of best evidence provides further direction for our work as educators.

SUMMARY

The teaching methods that we choose for our courses depend on our goals for learning. The classroom provides unique opportunities for learning with technology. Learning in a classroom setting is a revered and often

Exhibit 11.2

EVIDENCE-BASED REVIEW ABSTRACT: LISTENING FOR A "CLICK" IN CLASSROOMS

Compiled by: Shelley D. Barenklau, CRNA, MS

Audience response systems (ARS) using clicker remotes promote active learning and support classroom communication within a variety of academic settings. Clickers have entered classrooms to increase student participation, expand discussion, and challenge students to assess their level of understanding using an immediate feedback system. A literature review was conducted to examine best practice guidelines for implementing and utilizing ARS in graduate classrooms, specifically examining ARS use in nurse anesthesia education. A variety of goals and uses for ARS emerged from the review of the literature: increased classroom interactivity, inclusive classroom participation, promotion of attention spans, formative assessment, peer learning, and assessment of student accountability.

Overall, references suggest that clickers positively contribute to student comprehension, improved test scores, and satisfaction. Scientific conclusions for best practice guidelines for ARS are still emerging and further research is indicated as many existing references are experiential in nature. Clickers may prove to be a key to improving test scores or may be merely a fun and innovative method to capture student attention and generate classroom interaction. The answer remains a click away.

Bibliography

Cain, J., & Robinson, E. (2008). A primer on audience response systems: Current application and future consideration. *American Journal of Pharmaceutical Education, 72*(4), 1–6.

Caldwell, J. E. (2007). Clickers in the large classroom: Current research and best-practice tips. *Life Sciences Education, 6*(1), 9–20.

Collins, J. (2008). Audience response systems: Technology to engage learners. *Journal of the American College of Radiology, 5*(9), 993–1000.

DeBourgh, G. A. (2007). Use of classroom "clickers" to promote acquisition of advanced reasoning skills. *Nurse Education in Practice, 8*(2), 76–87.

Duncan, D., & Members of the Carl Wieman Science Education Initiative. (2009). *Clicker resource guide: An instructor's guide to the effective use of personal response systems (clickers) in teaching.* Retrieved October 16, 2009, from www.colorado.edu/sei/documents/clickeruse_guide0108.pdf

Duncan, D. (2008). *Tips for successful "clicker" use.* The Science Education Initiative, University of Colorado. Retrieved October 16, 2009, from www.colorado.edu/physics/Web/TipsforSuccessfulClickerUse.pdf

Institute of Medicine. (2003). *Health professions education: A bridge to quality.* Washington, DC: National Academies Press.

Jones, S., Henderson, D., & Sealover, P. (2009). "Clickers" in the classroom. *Teaching and Learning in Nursing, 4*(1), 2–5.

Martyn, M. (2007). Clickers in the classroom: An active learning approach. *Educause Quarterly, 2*, 1–6.

(Continued)

Exhibit 11.2

EVIDENCE-BASED REVIEW ABSTRACT: LISTENING FOR A "CLICK" IN CLASSROOMS (*Continued*)

Pradhan, A., Sparano, D., & Ananth, C. (2005). The influence of an audience re-sponse system on knowledge retention: An application to resident education. *American Journal of Obstetrics and Gynecology, 193*(5), 1827–1830.
Selen, M., & Stelzer, T. (2009). *The i-clicker top 10: Tips from our inventors.* Re-trieved October 16, 2009, from http://www.iclicker.com/dnn/LinkClick.aspx?fileticket=IM9s0cJ2KJM%3D&tabid=169

practical way to promote student knowledge gain. For many years faculty lectures, or telling students about content, has been the typical classroom approach. Now technology provides opportunities for enhanced learn-ing through interactive content applications. Technology in the changing classroom provides opportunities to combine the best of traditional and new teaching approaches.

ENDING REFLECTION

1. What is the most important content that you learned in this chapter?
2. What are your plans for using the information in this chapter in your future teaching endeavors?
3. What are your further learning goals?

GUIDELINES FOR THE CHANGING CLASSROOM AND TECHNOLOGY

Quick Tips for the Changing Classroom

1. Keep the classroom interactive with varied technologies such as clickers and pair/share activities.
2. If using PowerPoint, include reminder slides for interactive ac-tivities to break up a lecture.

3. Ask students to complete electronic fast feedback forms follow-
    ing class to indicate what they learned that was most useful and
    what they still have questions about.

Questions for Further Reflection

1. What makes the classroom unique for beginning students as com-
    pared to advanced students? Are there best practices for technol-
    ogy in the classroom depending on student level?
2. How can learning management systems best be used for the ped-
    agogical opportunities as well as management perspectives?

Learning Activity: Can PowerPoint Be Used for Active Learning?

Which of the following slides (or combinations) might help accomplish
student learning objectives for a class you plan to teach? Make a list of
those you would like to try using.

1. Specific slides that remind students what they have done to pre-
    pare for class (pre-assignments such as readings, pretests, or stu-
    dent reflections about their own experiences related to the topic)
2. Specific slides that remind you to create an introductory set for
    the class ("This is what we are going to accomplish today" or "Some
    of the things we will be doing include. . .")
3. Specific slides that remind you to include active learning oppor-
    tunities (PowerPoint slides that remind you to stop and engage
    students using techniques such as true/false questions, case stud-
    ies, pair/share activities, and other learning activities that help stu-
    dents engage with the content being taught, or a simple reminder
    slide with the word "questions?")
4. Preclass or postclass sharing of experiences or observations
5. Periodic summary slides ("So far this is what we've learned . . .")
6. A specific slide reminding you to bring closure to the lesson (for
    example, the high points covered)
7. A student "challenge" slide to consider how they might start using
    the content right away (additional assignments or a slide that sim-
    ply asks "What next?")

Online Resources for Further Learning

■ Classroom Assessment Techniques from the Field-tested Learning Assessment Guide (FLAG). A variety of assessment strategies that work well in student assessment with technology resources: http://www.flaguide.org/cat/cat.php

■ Preparing to Teach, Using Class Time Well. The University of Kansas Center for Teaching Excellence provides a variety of ideas and resources for making learning active in the classroom: http://www.cte.ku.edu/preparing/usingTime/

REFERENCES

Bailey, G. (1981). *Teacher self-assessment, a means for improving classroom instruction.* Washington, DC: National Education Association.

Bean, J. C. (1996). *Engaging ideas: The professor's guide to integrating writing, critical thinking, and active learning in the classroom.* San Francisco: Jossey-Bass.

Benner P. (2001). *From novice to expert, commemorative edition.* Upper Saddle River, NJ: Prentice Hall Health.

Benner P., Tanner, C., & Chesla, C. (2009). *Expertise in nursing practice: Caring, clinical judgment, and ethics* (2nd ed.). New York: Springer Publishing.

Bonnel, W., Fletcher, K., & Wingate, A. (2007). Integrating geriatric resources into the classroom, a virtual tour example. *Geriatric Nursing, 28*(5), 301–305.

Bradshaw, M., & Lowenstein, A. (2006). *Innovative teaching strategies in nursing and related health professions* (4th ed.). Sudbury, MA: Jones & Bartlett.

Bruff, D. (2009). *Teaching with classroom response systems: Creating active learning environments.* San Francisco: Jossey-Bass.

Commission on Behavioral and Social Sciences and Education. (1999). *How people learn: Bridging research and practice.* Washington, DC: The National Academies Press.

Fink, L. D. (2003). *Creating significant learning experiences: An integrated approach to designing college courses.* San Francisco: Jossey-Bass.

Institute of Medicine. (2003). *Health professions education: A bridge to quality.* Washington, DC: National Academies Press.

Malloch, K. (2009). Creating the context for technology: New realities for structure, media, space, and time. *Nursing Outlook, 57*(2), 116–118.

Rocklin, T. (1999). *PowerPoint is not evil.* Retrieved September 16, 2009, from http://www.ntlf.com/html/sf/notevil.htm

Skiba, D. (2008). Nursing education 2.0: Social networking for professionals. *Nursing Education Perspectives, 29*(6), 370–371.

Weimer, M. (2002). *Learner-centered teaching: Five key changes to practice.* San Francisco: Jossey-Bass.

Willis, B. (2004) *Distance education at a glance.* Retrieved September 18, 2009, from http://www.uiweb.uidaho.edu/eo/dist1.html

Simulation and Clinical Learning

CHAPTER GOAL

Gain a variety of ideas on how to incorporate simulation into students' clinical learning experiences.

BEGINNING REFLECTION

1. What experiences have you had with high-fidelity patient simulation (HFPS)?
2. What is your familiarity with gaming?

INTRODUCTION

How does technology relate to clinical learning? Because clinical practice is a fundamental element of nursing, teaching students to apply didactic content and skills to competent clinical practice is an essential element of their education. In the past, clinical skills were learned and practiced on live people. While that approach provided the necessary real-life experience, it also left concerns about the quality of care received by some patients, the ethical implications of practicing on people, and the problem that not all students had the same opportunity to experience the same clinical situations.

Advances in technology have led to methods that mitigate these concerns about clinical education. Students can now have virtual experiences that create the opportunity to learn a wide variety of specific clinical skills, as well as exercise the critical thinking skills necessary in live situations, without the potential risk of harming real patients. In these created situations or scenarios, students play the role of health care provider to simulated patients (a mannequin or computer character, for example) in fictitious settings (such as a hospital room, a hospital, or a community). Technology thus creates a means to provide clinical learning for all students that is safe, effective, and standardized.

In addition to creating a safer learning environment and standardizing clinical learning experiences for all students, simulation also provides opportunity for educational experiences based on best practices and sound educational theories. Being placed in a simulated scenario reinforces the immediate application of content suggested in adult education theory, the active participation of learners necessary to create meaning in constructivist theory, and the multiple intricacies of clinical situations in which students will actually practice as suggested in complexity theory. Although the exact technological means to do so will continue to change, two current examples of the use of simulation in health care education are HFPSs and electronic gaming.

HIGH-FIDELITY PATIENT SIMULATORS

Simulators are defined as "devices that attempt to recreate characteristics of the real world," and simulation fidelity is "the degree to which the simulator replicates reality" (Beaubien, 2009, p. 152). Low-fidelity simulators are not as lifelike as high-fidelity simulators. Perhaps the most basic simulators are the oranges into which many nursing students gave their first injections. As time progressed and mannequins were developed, students learned to give bed baths and provide range of motion exercises on mannequins. A few years later we were all learning cardiopulmonary resuscitation (CPR) on more sophisticated mannequins, which at least simulated a patient's general body and provided a mouth/nose and sternum on which to actually practice breathing and compression techniques. Some models also provide an electrocardiogram (EKG) strip to document the adequacy of (or lack thereof) the chest compressions. Today's

HFPSs, while still bearing a resemblance to the mannequins of days gone by, are much more refined, in that they blink, breathe, make urine, have EKGs and blood pressures and heart rhythms, and respond in physiologically appropriate ways to dose-specific medications. These mannequins come in infant, child, adult, and laboring women shapes and sizes.

The opportunities provided by these sophisticated machines are numerous. First of all, they provide a safe environment in which students can make mistakes without causing harm. Students can learn to critically analyze situations and either act appropriately or see the results of their mistakes and learn from that experience, without posing any danger to live patients. If a lethal dose of a medication is given to the simulated patient, he or she will "die." If the simulated patient's arrhythmia is treated incorrectly, he or she may "die."

Another advantage of simulators is that all students can experience the same clinical situations. Because the simulated experiences are fictitious, they can be created over and over again at any time, so that faculty and students are not dependent on what happens (or does not happen) at an actual clinical site. A faculty member who wants all students to run a code, or help with labor, or resuscitate an infant, can develop a scenario to match and use the HFPS to ensure that all students get that specific experience. Simulation offers not only an effective method by which to learn these lessons, but also an efficient method by which to evaluate students' formative and summative learning.

Potential Simulation Applications

In general, HFPS experiences are written as a patient situation in a clinical scenario, with students fulfilling various roles in the scenario. The scenario specifics are determined by the learning goals. There are a number of generic scenarios that can be purchased for a variety of clinical situations, but most of these scenarios need at least some revision to suit a specific learning experience.

For example, if you need to teach about do-not-resuscitate orders, then you might create a scenario in which a patient's heart and breathing stop, with this event serving as the catalyst for the scenario. Again, the content and courses in which scenarios can be used are almost limitless. For example, the HFPS might be used as a patient who needs the correct medication and dose for arthritis in a pharmacology course, a patient who needs to be coded in a critical care course, or a pediatric patient in a course teaching about asthma.

While the HFPS most often fills the patient role, students can play a variety of roles in the scenario. This area of best practices needs further attention, but, to date, there is little evidence to indicate whether the learning outcomes for students who observe the scenario and then participate in the debriefing are the same as those for students who actually play a role in the scenario and then participate in the debriefing. For example, students on site might actually play roles in the scenario, with the experience transmitted to distance students via live video streaming. Similarly, it is unclear if students must play the role of their chosen health profession in the scenario, or if the learning outcomes are comparable for students who might play a family member (rather than a doctor, nurse, pharmacist, or physical or occupation therapist) in the scenario.

It can be helpful to provide at least a little background on the characters students are to play in the scenario. Take, for example, a scenario in which four students will apply principles they learned in class about do-not-resuscitate orders. One student may play the nurse going off shift, another student may play the nurse coming on for the next shift, and two students might play children of the patient (the HFPS). At the outset of the simulation, each student would receive a short description of the character to be played. For example, the outgoing nurse would be given information about the patient's diagnosis, lab results, and vital signs to use in the report to the incoming nurse. The students playing children might be told that they are teenagers and that their terminally ill father has had cancer for years, and that they have agreed that no further intervention will be taken.

It is also helpful to have a number of events built into the scenario to help move the action along. For example, if the learning goal in the scenario is to apply the principles of do-not-resuscitate orders, then the scenario might start with the patient (the HFPS) in a room with his children (students). Shortly thereafter, the simulated patient would code, prompting two nurses (played by two students) to enter the room and initiate CPR. But the children (students) were told in their character descriptions that no further treatment would occur, so they would say, "Stop!" which would represent a decision point for the students playing the nurses. They might look around for the patient chart to confirm orders, find no do-not-resuscitate order, and determine that they must resume CPR. Any number of decision/action points can be created, and the nature of those decisions will depend on the learning goals.

Simulated experiences can be implemented in a variety of ways. For example, in some cases the faculty and students stop to discuss and plan their next steps with each change in the patient's status. This option has been used successfully, for example, in a critical care course and is very useful in helping students connect the didactic rationale to the clinical decisions they make. In addition to helping students apply critical thinking skills, with this approach faculty can choose to let students make mistakes or not. For example, students can become quite distraught if the simulated patient dies, and in some cases faculty may want to prevent that from happening by steering students toward more appropriate actions. On the other hand, if the learning goals are focused on learning about death and dying, or how to deal with poor outcomes, then it might be appropriate to let the patient "die" and help students work through their feelings.

In other classes, the simulated scenario unfolds in real time, with the students taking whatever action they think best, and the situation progressing accordingly (with the results—good or bad—depending on the student actions taken). For example, if a simulated patient is coded appropriately, he may live or die—just as live patients who are coded appropriately do, and that outcome may vary between groups of students. But if the students give a lethal dose of medication, the simulated patient will certainly "die."

Rubrics and Debriefing

As discussed in Chapter 9 ("Feedback, Debriefing, and Evaluation With Technology"), simulated experiences can be used for either feedback or evaluation. Whether formative or summative in nature, most simulated experiences are assessed according to a rubric that represents a criterion-referenced form of evaluation. Rubrics serve the dual purpose of providing a clear and precise guide both for students on the essential elements of the simulation and for faculty in assessing how well students achieve those essential elements. Rubrics should be as objective and measurable as possible. A simple rubric was provided in Chapter 9, but adaptations are likely required for each different scenario because of differing contexts (i.e., different courses, different learning goals, and different knowledge levels among students). For example, when making introductions, faculty might expect first-semester nursing students to merely state their name and title while making eye contact. But faculty might expect a senior nursing student to do that, as well as identify three items of patient assessment (i.e., level of consciousness, skin color/temperature, and heart rhythm on the monitor). In addition to the student criteria changing on the rubric, the faculty options for scoring might change. For example, if faculty let the scenario unfold according to the students' responses, then it is possible that an anticipated action may not occur; therefore the "not applicable" category in the rubric may be very appropriate. Also, as clear and distinct as we try to be with objective criteria, often unexpected events or variations occur, making the comments section indispensable. This section is also very helpful if more than one faculty member is assessing the same student, as rationale for different scores is important.

The debriefing session is held immediately after the simulation so that the memories of thought processes, actions, and feelings are still fresh. The session can be either faculty or student led, as long as all students are involved. Both general and specific questions are discussed. Some general debriefing questions were presented in Chapter 9, but, again, those questions need to be followed by more focused questions based on the specific learning goals. So, for example, in the previous do-not-resuscitate scenario, these additional questions might be asked:

1. What were you thinking when the patient coded and you decided to start CPR?
2. How did you feel when the children told you to stop CPR? How did that affect your actions?
3. I noticed you had trouble finding the patient's chart. Describe what was going through your mind during that time?

Advanced Simulations

The opportunities offered with simulations are increasing and expanding the options for using HFPSs in providing education. For example, simulators can be used in conjunction with other teaching modalities, such as standardized (paid) patients or electronic records. So, for example, in an interdisciplinary course focusing on intimate partner violence (IPV), a pediatric patient may be played by a pediatric HFPS, who presents in the emergency department with an asthma exacerbation. The patient's mother, who is the victim of IPV, might be played by a standardized patient.

Electronic health records (EHRs) could also be developed for this scenario, creating a history for this patient and his mother (rather than providing just the one-time glimpse into their lives represented by the scenario itself). In this way, the students could look back in the medical records and find frequent emergency department visits and other events suggestive of IPV in the family. Rather than the one-moment-in-time glimpse of a patient provided by simulation alone, the EHR provides a history in which the simulated patient has a past and a context in which to manage the simulated experience.

Questions to Ask Yourself

HFPS provides a unique means by which to engage students in active learning experiences within the safety of a lab setting. While cost once limited their availability, HFPSs are becoming increasingly available, if not in specific schools, at least regionally. However, as with so many teaching options, just because HFPS is available doesn't mean it is the best option. Guided by the Integrated Learning Triangle (Appendix B), consider the following as you think about using an HFPS experience:

1. What are the learning goals? Will a simulated experience help students achieve those goals?
2. What other teaching options are available that could also help students achieve the learning goals?
3. Which of the teaching options is the best fit? For example, if two options are considered equally effective in meeting the learning goals, the best fit is likely the least expensive, less time-consuming option. HFPSs are very expensive, as are their repairs, and so why risk overuse and damage to the simulator if a less expensive option is also available?
4. What support do you have for using the HFPS? While one faculty member may be sufficient to oversee the scenario, at the very least an additional staff/faculty member needs to be available to program and run the simulator. Also, is the simulator available when needed, or is it already booked for another class?
5. How will you achieve the learning goals if something prevents the HFPS from operating on a scheduled day? What other options are there for presenting this material as a backup plan?

An abstract of an evidence-based review, "Faculty Orientation to Learning Simulation," is shared at chapter end. This systematic review provides direction for developing faculty orientation programs for simulation.

ELECTRONIC GAMING

Children today are growing up with computer-based games and virtual worlds, and the opportunity exists to use that technology in health care education as well. These games are generally less familiar to more mature generations, but if you're under 30 years old or you have children/grandchildren under 30, then, whether or not you know it, you know electronic gaming.

Granted, much of the gaming may not be educational in nature, but it's gaming nonetheless. While many of the early games were for pure entertainment, their potential has now turned to the training of health care professionals, where students are immersed in real-life situations in which they must think and act accordingly. Second Life provides one gaming option in which virtual worlds, such as hospitals or even communities with clinics, can be created and in which the students can practice clinical and critical thinking skills.

Electronic games refer to interactive games provided via digital technology. While this definition includes today's pinball machines as well as new generation video games, electronic games also include elaborate virtual worlds. Serious games are further defined as those with an educational (rather than entertainment) purpose (Skiba, 2009a). While the concept may not be foreign to us, the idea of inserting ourselves—not as a generic game character but as a character using one's own thoughts, decisions, and actions—into that virtual world may feel less natural. Depending on the course, the virtual world may be a surgical suite, a hospital room, a medical center or long-term-care facility, a residential community, a city, a country, the world, or a completely alien world.

Whatever the virtual setting chosen, people in that setting are represented as avatars. An avatar is "a representation of oneself in a two- or three- dimensional world. Your avatar can be a character, person, or even an animal or icon" (Skiba, 2009b, p. 156). Electronic gaming is really a fairly natural extension of the human simulator. With HFPS the student him/herself is physically inserted into a scenario where he/she interacts with the patient and other health care providers; in gaming the student represents him/herself as an avatar and is inserted into a virtual world where he/she interacts virtually with the patient and other health care providers.

As with simulation, the options and opportunities with gaming are numerous. Gaming, too, provides a safe environment in which students can make mistakes without causing harm. Students can learn to critically analyze situations and either act appropriately or see the results of their mistakes and learn from that experience. Gaming can also be used to standardize clinical experiences for all students.

Potential Gaming Applications

While gaming provides many of the same options as simulation, it offers different strengths and weaknesses. For example, the simulated experience offers more lifelike interactions, and so, if interpersonal skills are included in the expected outcomes, then gaming may not be the best option available. However, if learning outcomes include learning about connecting patients with community resources, for example, then gaming may provide the better option. Gaming also offers the potential for synchronous and asynchronous interactions, and this convenience is often very attractive to students.

Rubrics and Debriefing

Many of the same principles regarding the use of rubrics and debriefing with simulation also apply to their use in gaming. Rubrics and debriefing can be helpful tools with gaming, and, in fact, the virtual world itself can be used for the debriefing session. Rubrics still provide a concise description of expected behaviors, but, if preferred, the actual clinical evaluation tool for a course could be used as the rubric for a gaming session. In any case, a set of objective outcomes that matches the learning goals is needed, as is the opportunity for students to discuss their performance and reactions to the experience.

Questions to Ask Yourself

As with HFPSs, just because gaming is available doesn't mean it is the best option. Guided by the Integrated Learning Triangle (Appendix B), ask yourself the same questions when trying to decide if gaming is the best teaching approach in a given situation:

1. What are the learning goals? Will a gaming experience help students achieve those goals?
2. What other teaching options are available that could also help students achieve the learning goals?
3. Which of the teaching options is the best fit? For example, if you are teaching cultural competence, students might be very engaged in a new, virtual culture that is different from any other culture they have ever experienced (if the faculty is very creative and develops a setting with entirely new creatures and customs and language). This option, however, will require a great deal of preparation time and effort, and, while it may teach valuable lessons, the actual customs learned won't have any real-world application

(because the faculty made the world up). Another option to teach the content might be to have a service learning project in which students go to a community center and care for elderly clients of a particular ethnic background. This experience might serve the same purpose of teaching valuable lessons about cultural competence, as well as actual customs that would have real world applicability, without using gaming at all.

4. How will you achieve the learning goals if something prevents you and the students from logging into the virtual space today? What other options are there for presenting this material as a backup plan?

HEALTH PROFESSIONS IMPLICATIONS

Simulated and gaming experiences provide the same advantages to health care providers who need to demonstrate new or ongoing proficiency on select clinical knowledge and skills as they do to the students. Many hospitals, for example, require that staff recertify on CPR and demonstrate competency in other skills on a regular basis. Similarly, education/demonstration experiences are required of staff as procedures and equipment are updated; simulated experiences may be an appropriate and efficient mechanism by which to teach and evaluate mastery of that knowledge and skills.

Along with the individual lessons, simulation offers one option by which to teach the interdisciplinary skills necessary to provide the quality care called for in the Institute of Medicine (IOM) reports. There are a number of competencies, for example, that are shared between medicine and nursing (such as communication, patient safety, and professional/ethical behavior), and both HFPS and gaming provide viable means by which students can gain interdisciplinary experience before providing that care to live patients.

INTEGRATED LEARNING TRIANGLE FOR TEACHING WITH TECHNOLOGIES

While falling most directly in the teaching/learning activities and feedback/assessment categories, the content about simulation and gaming in this chapter takes us all over the Triangle of Integrated Learning. Both are supported by educational theories and best practices. For example, through HFPS or Second Life, students actively participate in creating their own knowledge for immediate application, consistent with adult learning theory and constructivism.

The teaching/learning activities and feedback/assessment activities are guided most directly by the learning goals and objectives, and so that connection is strong. For example, if the students and/or hospital staff need to learn or recertify CPR, then a fairly basic mannequin will likely be used. Perhaps the school/hospital also owns a more sophisticated HFPS that could be used for the same experience. But if the learning goal is simply CPR and the lower-tech option is adequate to achieve the learning goals, then it may well be the better option as it respects the greater sophistication and delicacy of the more expensive HFPS, which is not needed to achieve the same goals.

Similarly, the teaching/learning and feedback/assessment options discussed in this chapter depend directly on situational factors. If your school or clinical site does not own or have access to an HFPS, then that is not an option. If you do not have a person with gaming expertise, who also has the time and interest to work with you, then gaming may not be a good option. So consider the available resources in terms of personnel, expertise, expense, time, and fit when deciding what technologies to use in a given situation.

Keep in mind that you, too, are part of the situational factors. Your commitment to lifelong learning will determine, in part, your willingness to try new teaching options. It will also affect the actions you do or don't take to seek resources beyond yourself and your institution.

For example, the National League of Nursing (NLN) offers a Simulation Innovation Resource Center (SIRC) online. This is an excellent resource for faculty both new to and experienced with HFPS. Further resources in developing and guiding simulations are also being published in journals and texts, including frameworks such as those provided by Jeffries (2007) and Nehring and Lashley (2009). Additionally, both HFPS and gaming are experiencing constant upgrades, so the literature changes rapidly, and both are ripe for new faculty who want to use, and/or contribute to, evidence-based best practices. Faculty need to be aware of their pivotal role in affecting the situational context.

As discussed previously in the chapter, the evidence-based review abstract "Faculty Orientation to Learning Simulation" is provided in Exhibit 12.1. This synthesis of best evidence provides further direction for our work as educators.

Exhibit 12.1

EVIDENCE-BASED REVIEW ABSTRACT: FACULTY ORIENTATION TO LEARNING SIMULATION

Compiled by: Christine L. Hober, MSN, RNC

Leaders in nursing education are implementing simulation for the interactive, collaborative, time-orientated experiential learning milieu that better prepares students for the real world of nursing. Simulation is known to engage the student in the scholarship of learning and teaching, while providing direction for clinical training utilizing the seven principles of best practice as discussed by Chickering and Gamson (1987). Simulation is a learning tool that requires technological knowledge and aptitude (Reeves, 2008). Research exposes that faculty have limited technological competence (King, Moseley, Hindenlang, & Kurtz, 2008).

This issue, coupled with nursing faculty shortages and national budgetary concerns, creates surmountable barriers to implementing simulation technology in practicum and theoretical venues. One possible solution is to facilitate the transition of faculty into simulation technology through structured orientation programs. This abstract synthesizes the literature for faculty orientation to infuse simulation into nursing curricula. Findings from the systematic literature review reveal that faculty simulation orientation programs need to be sustained over a period of time, be incorporated into faculty development plans, foster an open and invigorating informatics environment, connect accessible simulation mentors with faculty, and have institutional support (Curl, Smith, Chisholm, Hamilton, & McGee, 2007).

The research findings go on to show that informatic competencies must be infused into nursing curricula and faculty development plans in order to expand a nursing community of practice for prudent informatics technologies. This process can be augmented using Ajzen's theory of planned behavior (Sugar, Crawley, & Fine, 2004) and the STEP program (Jeffries, 2008). The STEP program recommends stages to bridging the gap of simulation technology with faculty development and curriculum innovations.

Essential factors to facilitate faculty ownership of simulation focus on providing: standardized materials easily accessible to faculty in a timely manner; ample time to train and retrain faculty; simulation design through integration teams; and ongoing simulation development and evaluation activities for faculty and students. Insightful research and lessons learned stress the applicability of simulation permeation using faculty expertise.

Ultimately, nursing educators will be taking a step toward best practices in nursing education while working toward high-quality patient care for the next generation of professional nurses by implementing simulation competence. As Jeffries (2007) suggested, simulation provides an opportunity for nurse educators to redesign educational programs to meet the needs of today's students.

Bibliography

Chickering, A. W., & Gamson, Z. F. (1987). Seven principles for good practice in undergraduate education. *The American Association for Higher Educa-*

(Continued)

Exhibit 12.1

EVIDENCE-BASED REVIEW ABSTRACT: FACULTY ORIENTATION TO LEARNING SIMULATION (*Continued*)

tion Bulletin. Retrieved February 28, 2009, from http://honolulu.hawaii. edu/intranet/committees/FacDevCom/guidebk/teachtip/7princip.htm

Curl, E. D., Smith, S., Chisholm, L., Hamilton, J., & McGee, L. A. (2007). Educational innovations. Multidimensional approaches to extending nurse faculty resources without testing faculty's patience. *Journal of Nursing Education, 46*(4), 193–195.

Jeffries, P. R. (2007). *Simulation in nursing education: From conceptualization to evaluation.* New York: National League of Nursing.

Jeffries, P. R. (2008). Simulations take educator preparation. *Nursing Education Perspectives, 29*(2), 70–73.

King, C. J., Moseley, S., Hindenlang, B., & Kurtz, P. (2008). Limited use of human patient simulation by nurse faculty: An intervention program designed to increase use. *International Journal of Nursing Education Scholarship, 5*(1), 1–17.

Reeves, K. (2008). Using simulated education for real learning. *MEDSURG Nursing, 17*(4), 219–220.

Sugar, W., Crawley, F., & Fine, B. (2004). Examining teachers' decisions to adopt new technology. *Educational Technology and Society, 7*(4), 201–213.

SUMMARY

Simulation offers a new and exciting method by which to teach health care professionals. Advantages include immersion in the real, though virtual, world, active learning, safety, and effectiveness. However, faculty need to use excellent critical thinking skills themselves to determine which simulated experiences are the best to use in any given situation.

ENDING REFLECTION

1. What is the most important content that you learned in this chapter?
2. What are your plans for using the information in this chapter in your future teaching endeavors?
3. What are your further learning goals?

GUIDELINES FOR SIMULATION AND CLINICAL LEARNING

Quick Tips

1. In a debriefing, be sure to include all students (with eye contact or by name, or both) equally if there are more students participating in the debriefing than participated in an actual scenario or game.

2. Consider using standardized case studies for simulation or gaming, especially if you're new to that technology. Don't hesitate to tailor the standardized case to your specific learning objectives.

3. Remember quality improvement approaches. As with most teaching activities, simulated or gaming experiences generally improve as they are continually revised and re-implemented in subsequent semesters.

Questions for Further Reflection

1. In many ways, simulations and gaming are merely extensions of the traditional case study. In what ways are the three similar and in what ways are they different?

2. Think of topics that you already teach, or plan to teach in the future. Do any of the topics lend themselves to simulation and/or gaming? On what rationale did you base your answers?

Learning Activity: Teaching Range of Motion

1. You have been assigned to teach the content on range of motion (ROM) to students. Consider and discuss the following:

    a. What would your learning goals be for the students?
    b. What would a ROM learning experience look like on a HFPS (describe the scenario, student roles, rubrics)?
    c. What would a ROM learning experience look like in Second Life (describe the virtual world, student roles, rubrics)?
    d. What other teaching methods could be used to teach the content?

    e. What aspects of the learning experience would you consider when deciding on the teaching method you would actually use to teach the ROM content?

    f. How would your activities change if you were evaluating students' ROM competency rather than teaching the ROM content?

Online Resources for Further Learning

- National League for Nursing, Simulation Innovation Resource Center. This site offers faculty a variety of online opportunities to learn about integrating simulation into nursing curricula: http://sirc.nln.org/
- International Nursing Association for Clinical Simulation and Learning. This site has tips for managing a simulation center, as well as links to numerous resource centers: http://inacsl.org/

REFERENCES

Beaubien, B. (2004). The use of simulation for training teamwork skills in health care: How low can you go? *Quality and Safety in Health Care, 13.* Retrieved October 10, 2009, from http://qshc.bmj.com/cgi/content/abstract/13/suppl_1/i51

Jeffries, P. (2007). *Simulation in nursing education: From conceptualization to evaluation.* New York: National League for Nursing.

Nehring, W., & Lashley, F. (2009). *High-fidelity patient simulation in nursing education.* Boston: Jones and Bartlett.

Skiba, D. J. (2009a). Emerging Technologies Center: Games for health. *Nursing Education Perspectives, 29*(4), 230–232.

Skiba, D. J. (2009b). Nursing education 2.0: Second Life. *Nursing Education Perspectives, 28*(3), 156–157.

13 Pedagogies, Technology, and Clinical Data Management

CHAPTER GOAL

Gain teaching/learning strategies to help students think critically and work responsibly with data and information systems.

BEGINNING REFLECTION

1. What are your experiences guiding students in learning about clinical data management and health information systems?
2. What further goals will help you and your students stay current with data management?

INTRODUCTION

Nursing students are preparing for a future where concepts of data management will be pervasive throughout clinical care. Students will be using technologies to gather and use data in assessing, planning, and evaluating individual patients. Teaching and learning broad concepts of data management in health care are central to safe, quality patient care. Helping students understand the basics of data collection and data management with a variety of patients, populations, and purposes is a key faculty role.

Pedagogy guides faculty in setting up lesson plans and clinical assignments to help students develop a skill set in data management. Guided by educational theories and best evidence, faculty can develop activities and assignments that promote ongoing student knowledge gain with data management as the central concept. Helping students learn to promote safe, efficient patient care using data management tools is an important faculty goal (American Association of Colleges of Nursing [AACN], 2008). Students learn decision making and critical thinking as part of informatics (McGonigle & Mastrian, 2008).

This chapter focuses on data management in clinical settings with information systems such as electronic health records to help students learn to provide quality care and promote patient safety. Concepts to be discussed related to information management and information systems include: the importance of this topic, opportunities for teaching and learning with electronic health records, varied teaching/learning opportunities specific to informatics, and broad curricular issues in nursing education.

THE IMPORTANCE OF TEACHING INFORMATION MANAGEMENT AND INFORMATION SYSTEMS

Data for decision making incorporate all aspects of health care. Informatics combines nursing science, information science, and computer science (McGonigle & Mastrian, 2008). Historically, clinical data have been handwritten on charts with information organized manually. The advent of computers and health information programs now provides opportunities for rapidly collecting and organizing even very large data sets. Now computers help clinicians assess and problem solve not only for an individual patient but also for large populations.

With the rapid advance of informatics in health care, a variety of professional organizations have confirmed the need for students to rapidly learn about informatics. These organizations also provide resources that can be used to assist and extend student learning. See Exhibit 13.1, "Examples of Organizations Supporting Informatics Education."

As a general guide, we want students to understand the benefits that information management and electronic information systems provide to a variety of entities including patients, health care professionals, consumers,

Exhibit 13.1

EXAMPLES OF ORGANIZATIONS SUPPORTING INFORMATICS EDUCATION

Understanding concepts of informatics and data management has been deemed critical by a variety of respected organizations. Sample organizations supporting integrating of informatics and providing resources include the following:

■ The National League for Nursing has published a position paper focusing on faculty preparation, "Preparing the Next Generation of Nurses to Practice in a Technology-Rich Environment: An Informatics Agenda": http://www.nln.org/aboutnln/PositionStatements/index.htm
■ The American Nurses Association has recognized informatics as a specialty for many years, maintaining the "Nursing Informatics: Scope and Standards of Practice" document, available at http://nursingworld.org/books/
■ AACN incorporates informatics competencies in its "Baccalaureate Essentials" document, discussing specific tools as well as the process of using informatics tools to promote safe, quality care, available at http://www.aacn.nche.edu/Education/bacessn.htm
■ The Institute of Medicine "Health Professions Educator Report" (2003) as well as various safety reports emphasize the need to educate the health professions in informatics: http://www.iom.edu/?id=12749
■ The Technology Informatics Guiding Educational Reform (TIGER) Initiative provides leadership on promoting informatics competencies in nursing programs as well as developing technology and informatics best practices for health professions: http://www.tigersummit.com/
■ The Robert Wood Johnson Foundation–funded Quality & Safety Education for Nurses (QSEN) project provides a repository for classroom assignments with relevance to several broad areas of health professions education: http://www.qsen.org/
■ Healthcare Information and Management Systems Society (HIMSS). This not-for-profit U.S. organization aims to promote better understanding of health care information and management systems: http://www.himss.org/ASP/index.asp

payers, and health care systems. Coeira (2003) summarized research supporting the following benefits to electronic information systems:

■ *Documentation for safe practice.* Preventing errors in patient care is a major concern, including not only clarity of written information but also enhanced communication among all responsible professionals.
■ *Quality improvement.* Providing quality care is enhanced by reflecting on information about practice. Electronic records provide

the opportunity for quality improvement, including data feedback mechanisms.

- *Patient self-care.* Patients ideally have opportunities for gaining their own electronic personal records that will be available wherever they seek health care; this provides care continuity as well as safety in clinical care.
- *Team communication.* Information systems (including electronic order entry, record keeping, and sharing of information between appropriate departments such as labs and pharmacies) promote team communication.
- *Decision support.* Rather than replacing decision making, electronic systems provide opportunities to monitor and support nurses' clinical decision making. Carty (2000) summarizes that electronic systems serve in a tutorial role for health professionals.
- *Monitoring.* Information systems provide opportunities for monitoring patient data and patient trends over time.

Information management consists of a number of related concepts. Information literacy and evidence-based practice, as discussed in earlier chapters, are intertwined with this topic. Computer literacy serves as just one component of informatics.

TEACHING AND LEARNING CRITICAL THINKING WITH ELECTRONIC HEALTH RECORDS AND DATA SETS

Learning with information management systems can help students learn to organize data. As all patients present with multiple, diverse symptoms, grouping patient data into patterns helps students make sense of the information. Informatics incorporates the complexity of patterns and helps organize or make sense of multiple pieces of data. For example, a patient's leg edema, shortness of breath, and weight gain are isolated facts for a new assessor. Electronic assessment forms support students' critical thinking skills to bring these data bits together as a pattern consistent with congestive heart failure. Students learn as individual patient data bits become patterns of information and then knowledge. Students learn about data being used in the following ways:

- To group data to first provide information and then to provide knowledge (whether for individual patients or large population groups)

- To follow outcomes-based practice via automated clinical pathways with databases to study care processes and outcomes
- To enhance clinical outcomes by decreasing errors—managing knowledge and information, making evidence-based decisions, and improving communication (IOM, 2001)

The Electronic Health Record as Learning Tool

The electronic health record has particular relevance in educating health professions students on both individual patient care and populations care. Carty (2000) notes that faculty use electronic health records to teach students judgment and information processing. The electronic health record is described as a legal record created in hospitals and ambulatory environments that serves as the central source of patient data (HIMSS, n.d.). Central elements of these tools specific to direct patient care include standardized forms with key terms and definitions that promote consistency in data collection.

In addition to clinical documentation and order entry, components of the electronic health record include clinical messaging, results reporting, data repository, and decision support (Hebda & Czar, 2008). The electronic health record also brings together information from a variety of departments, such as test results from laboratories and current medications from pharmacies. Information systems support clinical care delivery. They facilitate and transform data collection and use. The electronic health record, with its standardized terminology and templates, serves as a sample component of an electronic information management system and data set for student learning. Students gain in learning the following:

- Computers serve as tools in aggregating patient assessment data and then organizing data to identify a problem and develop a plan for patient care.
- Electronic records provide a type of electronic worksheet for gathering data and helping clarify and combine random facts in order to provide synthesized information.
- Students learn to think critically and manage information for patient problem solving and care planning using these tools.
- Students assess, record, and review patient data in practicing these skills.

- Students gain understanding of how separate pieces of data from assessments all come together for problem clarification and decision making.
- Information systems help collect and organize the data to help health care providers identify problems more efficiently for individual patients (as well as larger populations).

Standardized Electronic Forms as Communication Tools

Students gain clinical tools as they learn the benefits of the standardized assessment forms that electronic health records provide. In addition to gaining a baseline of assessment data on individual patients, these tools provide the following:

- Data for comparisons over time: Students learn that this information also helps compare patient progress over time. While providers have often monitored patients' status over time, oftentimes because of various health care system issues, access to clear comparison data for tracking patient progress was lacking.
- Reminder cues for thorough assessments: these tools provide cues that help students recall and avoid missing critical assessment questions. For example, when completing an assessment on a preoperative patient, cues provide reminders to question if a patient has a history of sleep apnea or has stopped specific medications—critical history questions. These electronic health record reminders also assist students in recording clear, concise, and complete information.
- Grouping of multiple individual's data: Students learn this information also helps describe populations and make comparisons across patient populations. For a beginning student assignment, patient data collected on standardized formats might be grouped and discussed in postconference.
- Accomplishing multiple tasks: Data collected on forms within electronic systems can be used specifically for both individual and population health. Additionally benefits to health care organizations exist in tracking selected data. The Long Term Care Minimum Data Set (MDS), a comprehensive system for electronic data management in long-term care, provides one example of how information systems can be used for multiple purposes.

Students see the implications of data use for individual patients. They begin to consider the benefits of understanding population data and the potential impact on care of groups of patients using standardized electronic data, comparing, for example, data on patients with diabetes.

Electronic Health Records as Tools for Care Planning

Standardized plans of care and resources for monitoring clinical pathways/outcomes are integral to the electronic health record and provide important student learning tools. Using electronic health records, once patient problems have been identified, decision support technologies can generate plans of care from evidence-based standards and protocols. Students then use critical thinking in confirming the appropriateness of the generated plan for a specified patient. As plans are implemented, information systems allow further monitoring of patients' progress. Consistency with clinical pathways and anticipated outcomes can be monitored. A common example of clinical pathways is use of core measures by hospitals on selected diagnoses to document quality care outcomes (The Joint Commission, 2009).

While clinical pathways provide broad, general patient care direction, clinicians' critical thinking is key in applying judgment to the patient's specific context. Additional critical thinking opportunities emerge for students when they care for patients with clinical problems that have not yet been well researched and developed into evidence-based protocols. As noted by McGonigle and Mastrian (2008), the whole point of information management is to support good decision making, the goal we have for our students.

VARIED TEACHING/LEARNING OPPORTUNITIES WITH ELECTRONIC INFORMATION SYSTEMS

Assignments can be developed around data sets to show implications for safe, quality patient care. Learning about clinical data sets helps students gain tools that have broad implications for patient care quality and safety. Assignments can be developed that help students relate or connect data specific to their individual patients to broader populations as well. Students can learn the importance of monitoring population variables to help document outcomes in our clinical units or agencies. Teaching quality improvement and population health are important opportunities with the electronic health record.

Teaching Continuous Quality Improvement

Data management systems allow new ways to help students think about projects such as quality improvement. Electronic health records allow not only easy access to collected data for individual patients but also opportunity to generate questions and compile data for a unit or population. An example of this quality improvement approach would include monitoring and studying information about variables related to clinical unit falls and adverse clinical events. While data sets are tools that nurses have used for years, their use has been limited because of the time-consuming manual manipulation of data. We used to have stacks of paper copies that recorded a unit's history of patient falls over a specified time frame. These might later be collated, but information analysis was at a distant point in time. New information management systems change this dynamic, allowing information to be compiled rapidly. Students can gain, sort, and learn about data for populations and groups as well as individuals. As faculty we can now help students use information management systems that provide more efficiency in quality assurance processes and lead to better, safer care for patients.

Teaching Population Health

Many opportunities exist for educators to use information management to help students learn about population problems. The following broad categories of informatics tools support public health: community health risk assessment (tools for knowledge acquisition; monitoring of disease outbreaks/epidemiology, and agency support), knowledge for health disaster planning and preparation, support of communication and dissemination to a population, and use of feedback to promote readiness and improve responses (McGonigle & Mastrian, 2008). Other topics include global public health disease surveillance and outbreak management. An assignment example includes gaining familiarity with local (and regional or national) public health informatics networks for managing outbreaks such as the flu.

Useful sites for teaching public health topics include the following:

- Centers for Disease Control (CDC)
- Healthy People 2020

- American Public Health Association
- Public Health Informatics (one of three centers within the CDC)
- Center for Public Health Informatics

While nursing educators are not expected to be experts in all public health arenas, a population focus is important to all. Networking with informatics nurse clinicians to gain speakers for classes and arrange student clinical experiences on these topics extends teaching/learning and practice opportunities.

CURRICULAR ISSUES FOR FURTHER THOUGHT

With the central role of informatics in health care, informatics becomes a curricular issue. One class on informatics is insufficient if similar content is not integrated across the curriculum. McBride (2005) notes that informatics competencies need to be implemented in all levels of nursing education. Diverse competencies have been proposed for health professionals. Many of these competencies take a novice to advanced practitioner approach. For example, beginning competencies in informatics have been described by Staggers, Gassert, and Curran (2002). The authors found that, in addition to basic computer competencies, novice health professionals needed informatics competencies related to categories of data, data impact, data privacy/security, and data systems.

There are new informatics roles for students to learn about. Students learn about staff roles in contributing to the development of electronic health systems and being part of the team. Information systems cannot be utilized in isolation. Systems theory states that all components of a system are interactive, so all team members will need to be well versed in these tools. Taxonomies and standardized language in particular have potential to enhance team communication about patient care among diverse providers and across disciplines. The AACN (2008) essentials document includes the need for students to be aware of their roles as team members as well as of the need for workflow attention and best design in electronic health systems. Students can learn the concept of participating as team members, advocating for designs that are both effective and efficient in patient care. Additionally attention draws to teaching informatics across diverse settings, considering inherent ethical/privacy issues, and considering further resources to support teaching informatics.

Understanding Informatics Variability Across Health Care Settings

Electronic health records are still evolving and vary by clinical sites. Many clinical sites still use unique systems, standards, and practices with limited communication across settings beyond the immediate practice. The black hole of patient documentation has been described by Thede (2009). Students need to be alert to the types of electronic documentation in a variety of settings. For example, in hospice settings there may be no electronic health records, although they may be needed. Many issues also exist around inconsistencies and cumbersome programs as health care systems seek to gain electronic health records. If there are different systems in different settings students will be working in, they need to understand the general concepts of electronic health records and then be prepared to adapt to alternate formats.

We may additionally be challenged to bring students up to speed, as many staff nurses are challenged themselves to gain data management expertise in new systems in their clinical agencies. A synthesis of the literature suggests both challenges and strategies for helping staff nurses gain competency. Suggestions include helping staff first gain competence in basic computer skills and then introduce more specific software and technologies (Collins, 2008). Awareness of this challenge and learning from staff development approaches may provide guidance for educators as well.

Ethical and Legal Issues

A variety of ethical issues related to data management exist that students need to know. Issues related to data management include the privacy rule and the Health Insurance Portability and Accountability Act (HIPAA). The privacy rule or standards for privacy of individually identifiable health information was issued to implement the requirements of the HIPAA (U.S. Department of Health and Human Services, 2003). The rule provides national standards regarding the disclosure of health information, seeking a balance between protecting individual's privacy and the flow of information needed to provide quality care. AACN (2008) makes clear that patient rights and ownership of the electronic health record are topics to be considered in nursing classrooms.

USING ELECTRONIC HEALTH RECORDS IN THE CLASSROOM

Opportunities exist for bringing electronic records to the students for learning in labs and classrooms. While in many schools students gain experience charting in electronic charts and records in clinical settings, some schools now provide this type of learning experience in their classroom and clinical lab settings. These systems can be used to create a wide range of fictitious patients, with many different medical issues, nursing needs, and personal/health care backgrounds. These records alone can be used to create a very complex patient for a case study or an entire unit of patients on which students can practice prioritizing critical thinking skills. In either case, these case records provide the context in which students see their "patients" and provide additional detail and history that can be used to develop students' critical thinking skills. Electronic records and the medical history can provide, for example, an entirely new dimension to the snapshot of a patient that students get during a simulated scenario. The SEEDS project (Warren, Meyer, Thompson, & Roche, in press) now teaches students, using created patient cases in the clinical lab, how to collect data, fill out standardized forms in created electronic charts, and then generate questions to identify potential patient problems. Projects such as SEEDS allow faculty to demonstrate first collection of data on individual patients and then data aggregation for the larger population.

Further Resources to Support Informatics Teaching/Learning

Various tools exist to help educators incorporate informatics into their teaching. Respected projects such as the Robert Wood Johnson Foundation–funded Quality & Safety Education for Nurses (QSEN) project provide specific student assignments relevant to informatics. Sample assignments include student self-assessments on informatics competencies as well as outlining how nurses use technology in their workplace (such as administration, communication, data access, documentation, client education, monitoring, quality improvement, and research).

Broad strategies such as expanding connections with clinical practice partners to include informatics speakers and opportunities for demonstrating system capabilities are recommended (National League for Nursing, 2008). AACN (2008) essentials recommend integrative student

Exhibit 13.2

LONG-TERM CARE MINIMUM DATA SET EXEMPLAR

The Minimum Data Set (MDS), used in long-term care nursing facilities, can serve as an example to help students understand the potential of electronic records in health care. Students can easily gain examples of the assessment tool and its uses from reputable, government-supported Web sites.

The MDS has a long-standing history as an information system and electronic health record in long-term care. The MDS standardized assessment tool is used to collect data on all nursing home residents, on admission and at specified intervals, as part of an electronic record. The recorded data then provides information used to monitor quality care indicators such as weight loss or depression for individual facility residents. For example, data from a facility resident who has been losing weight over a 3-month period will cause a flag on the electronic record, indicating that further attention to this problem is needed.

The information collected on individuals is then also combined to provide descriptive statistics on selected quality indicators for residents in the entire nursing home, state, or other geographic region. For example, a summary of the percentage of residents losing weight in one particular facility can be compared to percentages of residents losing weight in other facilities. Extensive data about specific nursing home resident variables can be gained when the right questions are asked of the MDS database. Reviewing the multiple uses for this tool with students can provide opportunity to begin discussions on electronic data management systems in general. Summary points include:

- At the resident level, the MDS includes basic resident assessment data completed on electronic records. These are called the resident assessment protocols (RAPs). These RAPs then serve to organize data for generation of a standardized care plan for specific residents.
- Nursing homes also transmit MDS data electronically to a state-based MDS repository. Information is then captured at the Centers for Medicare and Medicaid Services (CMS) national database. This information feeds into quality indicators as well as reimbursement guides at state and federal levels.
- This grouped resident data then also feeds into broad population information, allowing a type of benchmarking for long-term care facilities. Grouped resident assessment data on specific nursing home quality measures is posted at Nursing Home Compare (www.medicare.gov/nhcompare/). Each facility's data can then be compared to other facilities' data (making it possible to provide information about facilities, such as percentage of residents with weight loss or depression, to families).

learning experiences with a range of technologies to support patient care as well as student participation in quality assurance projects as a component of informatics.

Examples of Common Information Management Systems

Examples of standardized tools also are readily accessible on the Web. The Long Term Care Minimum Data Set is one example of an information management system with easy online access to data sets and information (see Exhibit 13.2). Faculty and students have ready access to learn about other data sets as well. For beginning students, introduction to large data sets could include well-recognized data sets. Examples of electronic data resources with Web resources and populations applications that might be used in classes include the following:

- The National Hospital Quality Measures (core measures), used by the Joint Commission on the Accreditation of Healthcare Organizations (JCAHO), to monitor hospital quality
- The National Database of Nursing Quality Indicators (NDNQI), maintained by the American Nurses Association, is used as a repository for nursing-sensitive indicators and outcomes (multiple hospitals submit data)
- The Functional Independence Measure (FIM) is the data set used to document disability and progress in rehabilitation settings
- The Outcome and Assessment Information Set (OASIS) is the data set used in home health care to assess and monitor home care clients.
- The Long Term Care Minimum Data Set (MDS) provides a comprehensive electronic record for use in long-term care facilities

Any of the above programs can be searched on the Web for summaries of their tools, processes, and outcomes. Having awareness of current approaches and where to learn more about these on the Web can be a good starting point for students.

SUMMARY

Clinical data management tools, such as electronic health records, are tools to enhance individual care within health care systems as well as tools to focus population care. Our goal is to gain tools/ideas for using technology with our students to promote student learning and ultimately safe, quality patient care. Students will continue to need more exposure and training related to information management systems at all levels of their education. In summary, we can help students learn in the following ways:

- Considering individual electronic data that students collect on their patients, including how collected data (individual bits) can be combined to create a holistic picture of patient needs
- Learning about how data can be grouped to provide knowledge of characteristics, activities, and outcomes of large populations
- Learning about evidence-based standardized plans that are patient relevant, students learn to follow outcomes-based practice via automated clinical pathways to study care processes and outcomes
- Focusing on accurate data recording, because this affects not only the patient record but also the facility record with issues such as payment and quality inspections
- Focusing on benefits of electronic health records with standardized data that can be tracked over time and shared with multiple providers
- Using data at advanced student levels for answering evaluative and research questions

While the tools we use will be changing, broad teaching learning principles assist students in gaining comfort with basic concepts and changing technologies. Health professions educators have the responsibility to prepare students of the future with a variety of tools that make them effective practitioners and team members. Changing technologies will be their tools as they work with patients for safe, effective quality care.

ENDING REFLECTION

1. What is the most important content that you learned in this chapter?
2. What are your plans for using the information in this chapter in your future teaching endeavors?
3. What are your further learning goals?

GUIDELINES FOR PEDAGOGIES, TECHNOLOGY, AND CLINICAL DATA MANAGEMENT

Quick Tips for Clinical Data Management

1. Think about the varied ways electronic data is used in a familiar clinical agency and use these exemplars with students.
2. Help students learn about population health using online resources such as Healthy People 2020 in creating assignments.
3. Talk with clinical partners about their quality improvement projects to help students gain exemplars of data management for improved patient care.

Questions for Further Reflection

1. What are the best strategies for training students on multiple electronic record systems when there is limited clinical time?
2. What are best practices in using information systems to assist students in promoting safe, quality patient care?

Learning Activity

Make a list of the ways that you use information management in working with students in clinical settings. Do these activities or assignments include topics related to administration, communication, data access, documentation, education, monitoring? Use software and systems? Are there ways these approaches could be expanded?

Online Resources for Further Learning

- TIGER Initiative (Health Information Technology). The TIGER competencies and suggested targets for knowledge, skill, and attitude development during prelicensure education are provided: http://www.tigersummit.com/
- Quality & Safety Education for Nurses (QSEN). This Web site provides extensive resources and sample assignments organized around safety, quality, and the additional recommended competencies of the IOM (2003) Health Professions Report including informatics: http://www.qsen.org/

REFERENCES

American Association of Colleges of Nursing. (2008). *The essentials of baccalaureate education for professional nursing practice.* Retrieved September 20, 2009, from http://www.aacn.nche.edu/Education/bacessn.htm

Carty, B. (2000). *Nursing informatics: Education for practice* (2nd ed.). New York: Springer Publishing.

Coeira, E. (2003). *Guide to health informatics* (2nd ed.). Great Britain: Hodder Arnold Publication.

Collins, M. (2008). *Best practices to facilitate adoption of computerized information systems among older nurses.* Unpublished paper, University of Kansas School of Nursing.

Hebda, T., & Czar, P. (2008). *Handbook of informatics for nurses and health care professionals.* Saddle River, NJ: Prentice Hall

Healthcare Information and Management Systems Society. (n.d.). *The electronic health record.* Retrieved October 16, 2009, from http://www.himss.org/ASP/index.asp

Institute of Medicine (IOM). (2001). *Crossing the quality chasm.* Washington, DC: National Academies Press.

Institute of Medicine (IOM). (2003). *Health professions education: A bridge to quality.* Washington, DC: National Academies Press.

The Joint Commission. (2009). *Performance measurement initiatives.* Retrieved October 16, 2009, from http://www.jointcommission.org/PerformanceMeasurement/PerformanceMeasurement/

McBride, A. B. (2005). Nursing and the informatics revolution. *Nursing Outlook, 53*(4), 183–191.

McGonigle, D., & Mastrian, K. (2008). *Nursing informatics and the foundation of knowledge.* Boston, MA: Jones & Bartlett Publishers.

National League for Nursing. (2008). *Preparing the next generation of nurses to practice in a technology-rich environment: An informatics agenda.* Retrieved September 20, 2009, from http://www.nln.org/aboutnln/PositionStatements/index.htm

Staggers, N., Gassert, C., & Curran, C. (2002). A delphi study to determine informatics competencies for nurses at four levels of practice. *Nursing Research, 51,* 383–390.

Thede, L., & Sewell, J. (2009). *Informatics and nursing: Competencies and applications.* Philadelphia: Lippincott.

U.S. Department of Health and Human Services. (2003). *Summary of the HIPAA privacy rule.* Retrieved October 12, 2009, from http://www.hhs.gov/ocr/privacy/hipaa/understanding/summary/index.html

Warren, J., Meyer, M., Thompson, T., & Roche, A. (in press). Transforming nursing education: Integrating informatics and simulations. In C. Weaver, C. Delaney, P. Weber, & R. Carr (Eds.), *Nursing and informatics for the 21st century: An international look at practice, trends and the future* (2nd ed.). Chicago: Healthcare Information and Management Systems Society.

14 Pedagogy, Technology, and Clinical Education

CHAPTER GOAL

To use technologies in preparing students to provide safe, quality care in clinical settings.

BEGINNING REFLECTION

1. What experiences (as an educator or student) have you had using technology in the clinical setting?
2. What are examples of your best and most challenging experiences?

INTRODUCTION

Clinical experiences are central in creating nursing providers. Health care education has always been distinguished in preparing students to care for patients in actual clinical settings. This unique clinical practice brings many opportunities and challenges in using technology when working with students. A number of Institute of Medicine (IOM) safety reports have made clear that faculty need to play a major role in developing safe students for the clinical setting. Technology has been identified as a central tool to promoting safe, quality patient care and supporting a clinical culture of safety (IOM, Committee on the Health Professions Education, 2003).

As new technologies have emerged for both clinical labs and actual clinical care settings, more opportunities to develop optimal pedagogy and technology combinations exist. In the past, students went to the classroom and clinical practicums with limited technology resources for learning. Now students have access to numerous electronic books and Web resources in preparing for clinical patient care. In the past, faculty often prepared students for their clinical experiences with some role-play type activity in the clinical lab rather than with the high-fidelity patient simulator or virtual gaming that now presents opportunities for learning safe clinical practice. We now have opportunities to be creative with a variety of technology resources in learning what works best to develop safe practitioners.

Knowledge gained in the classroom needs to be applied in clinical settings while keeping patients safe and effectively cared for. This chapter helps us think about how best to use technology in organizing teaching for our clinically focused outcomes. As changes occur in both clinical labs and the hospital setting, how can technology assist faculty in developing safe health care professionals? This chapter discusses pedagogies to support technology as a tool in the changing clinical labs and in the clinical units and agencies. It also discusses technology as a tool for caring for patients at the point of care. Finally, the role of telehealth in caregiving at a distance is considered.

PEDAGOGY AND THE CHANGING CLINICAL LEARNING LAB

The clinical laboratory provides a structured teaching environment in which students can learn safe application of skills as well as critical thinking. The clinical lab has been described as a resource for multiple health providers (Hudson-Carlton & Worrell-Carlisle, 2005) offering a variety of teaching/learning opportunities. Teaching devices range from simple mannequins to electronic arms for practicing intravenous injection to authentically simulated patients. Practice labs provide opportunities for students to gain comfort with a variety of challenging skills such as intravenous starts, nasogastric tube insertion, intubation, and blood administration. The learning lab takes on new importance with access to high-fidelity patient simulations that provide students real-time practice in intense or high-risk situations that would be limited in the real-world clinical setting.

Learning labs are unique settings with tools and resources that vary by school from low- to high-technology sites. Some labs mimic hospital settings in appearance and others include clinic rooms and home-based simulations. In many, the high-fidelity patient simulators have become important tools and have led to whole families of simulators in the learning lab. Galloway (2009) provides an extensive discussion of the types of simulator technologies to be found in the learning lab that provide students with safe practice and learning opportunities.

The pedagogy of clinical teaching incorporates applied learning. Consistent with classroom teaching, faculty assess learners' needs and match assignments to class objectives, focusing on the interactive learning opportunities available in the lab setting. We identify students' strengths and weaknesses, as well as provide assignments that promote practice and build student confidence and safety. Clinical learning labs also provide opportunities for increased focus on self-directed learning and documentation of student competencies.

How do faculty best use technology to organize effective clinical preparation experiences that prepare students for safe clinical practice? Questions to consider for the clinical lab include the following:

- What are the benefits of lab practice? How much practice and how much "actual" clinical experience are needed?
- What do we mean by "student practice" and how will it be structured?
- How many ways are there to help students learn with technology in the learning lab? How real and safe can faculty make those experiences?
- What are the requirements for student preparation to come to the learning lab? How prepared should faculty expect students to be before walking in the lab door?

The clinical learning lab can provide a functional, supportive environment for learning. To be effective and efficient, attention must be paid to the design of the setting of the learning activities, and to the support staff in the lab (from faculty to teaching assistants). All of these individuals must use good principles of teaching and learning as they work with students on clinical lab assignments. Sample approaches to promote success in the clinical lab, no matter what the technology to be used, include orienting students to their roles, clearly identifying lab purposes, and determining rubrics to guide learning.

Orienting Students to Clinical Lab Learning Assignments

Faculty can help students understand the expectations for each clinical lab assignment by guiding students in preparation for the lab. This includes clarity on preparation expectations, including reading assignments and practice activities prior to the lab assignment. In the past we used class time to watch video and practice in the lab. Now if we choose, we can have students "pre-watch" an orientation online. Prepping for the clinical lab becomes a new experience with the variety of teaching and learning aids available online. While benefits exist to these online resources, potential challenges also exist if students seek their own Web resources that may not have been critiqued or peer reviewed. Appropriate guidelines for Web resource review then become a part of clinical learning orientation.

Ideally the students come to the lab ready to apply what they have read ahead of time, and have more time to apply knowledge and work on the skills. Even having learning activities such as PDA-based assignments available for dealing with downtime while students are waiting to be checked off on a skill promotes use of learning time.

Identifying Lab Purposes and Effective Assignment Design

In terms of overall lab planning, setting specific objectives for learning lab sessions is central. Effective lab assignments are guided by session objectives. Guided by the Integrated Learning Triangle (Appendix B), concepts of assessment, appropriate learning activities, and evaluation come together. Determining if the learning lab assignment is for practice and learning or whether it will include a summative grade is considered in the planning phase. Walvoord and Anderson (1998) note the importance of this determination and students' awareness prior to evaluation. How is technology best used to help with lab check-offs and for monitoring student progression?

- Is the lab time scheduled with faculty available to provide instruction as students practice?
- Is the lab time a student solo effort or do students assist each other with assigned roles?
- Are procedure check-offs required? Are students required to share the theory/rationale that supports the behaviors they demonstrate?
- Are check-offs completed by faculty or a teaching assistant? Are check-offs completed by peers acceptable? Can self-assessment and peer review be part of check-offs?
- Are lab check-offs just skills checklists or do they include making a "chart note" related to the case study/clinical skill? There are advantages to having students access computers and learn recording procedures/charting on electronic health records as they will be doing in most actual clinical settings (Warren, Meyer, Thompson, & Roche, in press).

Guiding Labs With Clinical Rubrics and Checklists

Rubrics or checklists are beneficial in both facilitating the lab experience and the clinical grading for faculty and students. They promote clear communication as to expectations of best practice in completing skills. Providing skills checklists for students provides direction in their skill learning and practice. Students can use these tools for self-assessments and participate in peer assessments to promote learning.

Since there can be differences in how these forms are interpreted when these tools are used by multiple faculty for evaluation, gaining interrater reliability is important to promote fairness in evaluation. Within learning management systems, these checklists can be distributed to students, as well as checked off, and tracked or monitored for competencies. Some of the noted check-off questions are curricular discussions and will include discussion of rubrics or tools that faculty teams need to address.

Using Technology to Plan Clinical Experiences

The clinical setting is complex with busy staff, anxious students, and often complicated patient care. For clinical staff there may be challenges working with students related to multiple schools, varied levels of students, varied assignments, and a variety of staff and health professionals. Helping staff in the clinical settings better understand faculty plans and student needs provides a good start to the clinical experience. Thinking about clinical education as a linkage between education and practice can promote ease of planning. Technology can be used for sharing clinical resources. Benefits exist for a central online resource for housing orientation materials that staff as well as students can access. Web sites can be used to facilitate the clinical experiences in the following ways:

- ■ *Initial organizing.* Many schools and hospitals have formed partnerships, using the Web as a tool for scheduling students, to promote optimal student numbers for patient care.
- ■ *Document repository.* Web sites provide spots for housing the clinical learning documents, evaluation guidelines, and student rosters with needed information.
- ■ *Ongoing communication.* Providing online access to clinical tools for staff and preceptors can not only promote ease in accessing student resources but also enhance communication with clinicians.

Sharing needed clinical tools and accessing preceptors using technology serves as a way to promote team communication. An example of an online studio developed for doctorate of nursing practice (DNP) preceptors is described in Exhibit 14.1.

Exhibit 14.1

CASE EXAMPLE: ONLINE DNP PRECEPTOR STUDIO

Compiled by: Diane Ebbert, PhD, ARNP, FNP-BC, and Moya Peterson, RN, MS, CPNP, ARNP, PhD

The importance of well-prepared preceptors in socializing advanced practice nursing students is clear. While DNP programs are being developed by various schools and organizations, preceptor training of DNPs has not been well addressed. This case example describes the Online DNP Preceptor Studio, part of a new DNP postmaster's program at University of Kansas. Donabedien's framework of structure, process, and outcomes organized the development of this studio. The Preceptor Studio, a new Web-based resource, is designed to assist advance practice preceptors gain or update teaching skills.

The structure of the resource (including the studio format and available preceptor resources); the studio development process (including focus group data from practitioners); and outcomes (beginning evaluative data including preceptor use of resources, self-assessment scores, and studio/resource satisfaction) are shared

(Continued)

Exhibit 14.1

CASE EXAMPLE: ONLINE DNP PRECEPTOR STUDIO (*Continued*)

online. Adult education principles, evidence-based practices from multiple disciplines, and National Organization of Nurse Practitioner Faculty inform the precepting resources. Tools such as best practice tools for personal digital assistants (PDAs), Web-based resources for fingertip knowledge, and resources for coaching and mentoring are part of this resource. The online studio is unique in preparing the much-needed clinicians/preceptors for applying evidence-based practice at the bedside and gaining coping skills in new preceptor roles. This just-in-time learning resource provides tools and ideas useful in other programs as well.

Faculty Orientation to Clinical Units and Technology

As faculty preparing to take students to clinical units, we want to be as familiar as possible with these settings. Gaining familiarity includes exploring the clinical unit and determining the learning team participants (clinical facility staff, instructors, students, patients, and college partners). Reviewing clinical unit Web resources and having needed names and contact information available electronically promotes ease of communication. Technologies can provide faculty support in gaining familiarity with clinical units and organizing the first days of class and clinical experiences, additionally providing opportunities to engage staff as partners in educating our clinical students. Sample technology considerations for clinical faculty include the following:

- What broad technology resources and tools will be used by students? For example, what technologies will be used for medication administration and accessing the medication system?
- What electronic health records are used and what system is used for students to access needed records?

Student Orientations

Beginning a clinical experience involves setting a positive climate for student learning, both physically and emotionally. Helping students move from clinical lab technologies to hands-on caring is a key faculty endeavor. The goals are to help students gain comfort, increase skills, and be safe in the clinical setting. Orienting students to their roles and the setting is important in helping them gain comfort, thus minimizing their anxiety as they begin their clinical learning. In a given clinical setting, technology can help organize an effective orientation organized around the important concepts of place, people, and process. Help students consider each of these concepts—the physical structure and resources of an emergency room, the process and protocols for providing care, and the expected patient outcomes and how these are documented.

- ***The Place.*** Orientation to place involves gaining familiarity with and comfort in the physical environment, including the layout and the resources. Can electronic documents be distributed to students that will promote way finding? Can videos of units be shown to provide an introductory orientation? Are in-house electronic resources available that provide students information about the laboratory, diagnostic, and pharmacy resources?
- ***The Process.*** Orientation to the process involves identifying how things are done on the unit and how students can participate. Are selected staff willing to provide a brief welcome video to students, sharing their philosophy of the clinical unit?
- ***The People.*** Orientation to people means being introduced to key staff that students will be working with. Are there electronic repositories with staff introductions or professional social networks students can use to gain introductions?

The clinical syllabus serves as an orientation tool and can be outlined and shared electronically with students as well as staff. Additional ideas for orienting students include: electronic introductory letters (to both students and staff), tours (video or face-to-face), and scavenger hunts (electronic or face-to-face).

Facilitating and Supervising Work With Students

The clinical setting brings new challenges to address as students bring their own anxieties and stresses to busy, complex clinical units with diverse patient needs. As students move into the actual clinical setting, our goal is to integrate technology and other resources for promoting student and patient clinical safety, building on what students learned in the clinical lab. How do faculty keep up with their many students and their patients' medications, treatments, diagnostic tests, and clinical procedures? Beginning approaches include using technology, such as in the following ways, to plan clinical experiences:

- Online resources or electronic distribution of resource materials
- Web-based tools to access students' postclinical write-ups or reflective journals
- Online discussions for postclinical sharing and debriefing
- Electronic management systems, including tracking systems, such as Typhon, that track the types of patient care experiences that students have had and generate reports that summarize cumulative clinical experiences

What is the best way to keep track of students who are correlating content for critical thinking and safe care of patients? Coaching and supervising students using technology includes maintaining good communication with students. This process often involves issues with multiple units and communications with both students and resource clinicians. Technology provides help such as increased access to preceptors, PDAs for clinical logs, and technology through which students can check in and follow up with faculty.

PDAs or mobile computing devices are efficient tools for faculty organization. This technology, a type of automated notebook or clipboard, serves as an organizing tool for faculty to support supervision responsibilities. Examples of ways that mobile computing devices such as PDAs can help faculty organize include the following:

- Electronic assignment grids for organizing clinical days with students
- Reminder systems for tracking students and procedures
- Tools for quick clinical notes such as student anecdotal records

PDAs also serve as information resources to guide students in evidence-based practice, providing students access to portable texts and online resources to maintain convenient access to an evidence base for confirming plans and approaches. Particularly as students learn new medications, these tools help to confirm dosages, alerting students to potential problems or side effects of medical orders. This clinical technology has benefits to patient safety as well as advantages to convenience in organizing large amounts of information. New uses of video with these pocket type devices are also being developed. Exhibit 14.2 provides a case example using Pocit Videos. Additionally, the Health Insurance Portability and Accountability Act (HIPAA) privacy issues in clinical settings and the need for PDA password protection are noted.

Exhibit 14.2

CASE EXAMPLE: POCIT VIDEOS: POINT-OF-CARE INSTANT TEACHER

Compiled by: Mary N. Meyer, RN, MSN, ARNP, and Sharon Kumm, RN, MN, CCRN

In a rapidly changing clinical environment, students are faced with multiple ways of doing basic procedures. While procedures change in response to new research findings, change at the bedside may lag behind the evidence. To complicate matters, there is frequently more than one *correct* way to perform basic nursing procedures. Even when students accept more than one "right way" as acceptable, students are frustrated when teaching is inconsistent.

Requiring PDAs for our undergraduate nursing students for the past several years, we wanted to expand their learning opportunities beyond the traditional textbooks. A faculty member proposed the idea of producing digital videos of techniques that could be placed on the PDA for students to review in clinical settings. In addition to providing the students instant access to best practice, the videos might encourage the student to share the best practice with staff nurses or use the videos as a patient teaching aide. After a faculty and student survey as to the most needed videos was conducted, five videos varying from tracheostomy care to insertion of intravenous catheters were developed. The process for video development included: use of current evidence from the literature for script development; graduate teaching assistants volunteered to be the actors; and the institution's instructional support department assisted with filming, voice over, and editing the digital product. Videos were stored on the online learning management system, allowing students to access and download them from several courses. Faculty encouraged students to access the videos.

After project implementation the first semester, approval was gained from the institution's institutional review board for a student and faculty survey on project satisfaction. With the exception of wanting more orientation to accessing the videos, other comments were favorable as to satisfaction with the videos. This project is ongoing and was developed with support from the National League for Nursing (NLN) Health Information Technology Scholars (HITS) program.

Technology and Documenting for Learning

Clinical care and documentation are intertwined. Critical thinking is enhanced as students determine what information to pass on to their patient team. Technologies can help in orienting students to clinical preparation and documentation expectations. The following questions can guide thinking about particular pedagogies:

- What type of preparation sheets, care plans, or concept maps will students be completing on assigned patients? What questions should they be prepared to answer for evidence-based care? What technologies can support their work in these areas?

- How are students best prepared to communicate with the team? What ways are students best challenged to gain skill with the situation-background-assessment-recommendation (SBAR) technique? How does this help prepare for electronic documentation?
- What documentation systems will students be utilizing in working with their patients? What guidelines do students need? Electronic health records as discussed in Chapter 13 are a central part of learning.

Conferencing and Debriefing

The purpose of the postclinical conference is to debrief and assist students in reflecting on and learning from their experiences. The reflection on practice or reflective practice that a postclinical debriefing allows fits well with technologies. Literature on simulations has highlighted the importance of these postclinical debriefings (Jeffries, 2007).

Arranging mutual times and locations for postclinical conferences can be challenging. Using electronic methods can ease this challenge, with online resources providing an alternate approach to traditional face-to-face clinical conferencing. Technology can help here in the following ways:

- Debriefing online can include student journals or clinical day summaries completed electronically and shared with faculty via electronic methods such as e-mail or learning management systems.
- Clinical narratives based on Benner's model (Benner, Hooper-Kyriakidis, & Stannard, 1999) shared in electronic portfolio format provide students with an opportunity to name what they are doing. Using precourse and then postcourse narratives encourages students to note their advancing skills (seeking higher-order practice across the semester).
- Preconferences can also use technology to help assess learner readiness and help learners prioritize their learning needs/goals. Faculty might conduct preconferences online when necessary.

Using Technologies in Clinical Evaluation

Clinical evaluation is enhanced by technology. Once faculty have organized a good clinical experience for students, technology can help provide clinical feedback on written work, patient care observations, or even distant site clinical experiences. Broad evaluation concepts are described in Chapter 9 and build on the American Association of Higher Education Assessment Forum (1993) guidelines. These guidelines include specific approaches and rationale for tools used to evaluate students' work, such as evaluative data that combine reflections, written work/exams, and clinical observations and involve multiple reviewers when possible. Technology can help with the following:

- Triangulating of evaluation methods and evaluators, with increased use of clinical learning labs in competency checks
- Tracking of minimum safety competencies checked off in the learning lab
- Making best uses of clinical rubrics for evaluation of student written work
- Amassing multiple sources of data for evaluation: student report, patient report, staff report, observation, and record review
- Developing student skills in self-assessment and peer review (e.g., students may do self-assessments and peer check-offs against a rubric as practice for a final)
- Completing summative evaluations with input from the learner (e.g., inviting the learner's self-assessment in electronic format, comparing this to faculty summation, and using any differences as points for further discussion)
- Sharing electronic preceptor evaluation and site evaluation tools for students to complete

Clinical tracking systems, as noted earlier, exist in which students' clinical experiences, the number of hours spent, preceptors used, facilities visited, and objectives met can all be logged and documented. These systems can track students across their entire academic programs, documenting the types of patients they see, the procedures they complete, and their progress from course to course. They simplify record keeping and save faculty time as well.

TECHNOLOGIES FOR ASSISTING PATIENTS AT POINT OF CARE

Technologies are pervasive in clinical care. Devices are as basic as electronic thermometers and blood pressure devices purchased at local drug stores. Clinical technology tools can include telephones for verbal monitoring of patient progress and digital cameras to monitor wound progression. Guiding and evaluating students in technology-rich clinical settings are central faculty roles. At the point of care there are all kinds of technologies for students to gain comfort with. Students are introduced to devices that translate patients' basic physiologic functions to screens and printouts for monitoring patient care. From monitors to tubes and central lines, the opportunities for learning with technology are extensive. The American Association of Colleges of Nursing (AACN) essentials specifically address the need for student learning about applications of clinical care technology (AACN, 2008).

Critical care and surgical care settings provide good examples of extensive technologies for monitoring patients and supporting their care needs. Even general hospital units often resemble the critical care units of years past. Technologies are key features in home care as well. Technologies that support patient care include patient monitoring equipment, drug and IV system alerts, and patient identification systems such as bar coding. They are therefore considered essential in nursing education (AACN, 2008). At the point of care there are numerous technologies for students to gain comfort with.

All tools are new to students at some point, including technologies such as cardiac monitors and respirators that have been a part of clinical experiences for many years. In getting our students ready for the work world, basic approaches to teaching these technologies can begin in the clinical lab. For all types of technology, students need to know the basic purposes, how to monitor for correct function, and how to troubleshoot problems. Students gain comfort with the technology "parts" as well as the evidence-based protocols that guide their use.

Safe and prudent use of technology includes practical technology assessments (Benner et al., 1999). In their discussion of technology in the critical care setting, Benner et al. note that practical technology assessments include determination of its usefulness for a particular patient, safety factors, accurate management, and for interpreting equipment performance readings correctly. The authors described ethical considerations in technology as well as its safe use. In addition to learning how a particular technology works and how to interpret the data provided, students will need to consider how to blend caring and direct hands-on care (high touch) with technologies. Students are reminded how important it is to care for the patient and not focus just on the technologies.

While not all new nurses will specialize in clinical areas where patient care technology is extensive, opportunities exist for all students to learn the basics of safe, reasonable care according to standards. As graduates seek to specialize, the tools they have gained as lifelong learners can help them with ongoing technology updates.

Faculty can create introductory assignments that allow students to gain comfort with a range of technologies. For example, faculty could start a class by asking students to brainstorm how many ways they use technologies in patient care. Then extend the discussion to include questions that help students address the benefits and challenges of selected technologies. Exhibit 14.3 suggests sample assignments for enhancing technology awareness in the clinical setting.

Exhibit 14.3

SAMPLE ASSIGNMENTS FOR ENHANCING TECHNOLOGY AWARENESS IN THE CLINICAL SETTING

- Ask students to brainstorm types of technologies patients/families can purchase at the local drugstore, such as basic electronic thermometers and blood pressure devices.
- Ask students to think of times they have used technologies as monitoring devices, such as pulse oximetry or EKG rhythm strips.
- Ask students to review online product resources, both written and video, to prepare for their clinical experiences.
- Have students make a survey of the tools/technologies they will be using in a clinical rotation, such as central line transducers, ventilators, fetal monitoring equipment, or remote telemetry. Include Web resources that provide product reviews, or divide students into groups and ask them to share a product summary from the Web.
- Use the Web for clinical preparation. Students learn new clinical technologies by reviewing online product resources, both written and video. Hermann (2009) describes the "equipment conference" where students focus on learning the mechanics and the clinician role in using technologies that are new to them.
- Assign students to work with expert staff and observe these tools being used efficiently and appropriately.
- Consider electronic medication management issues, including topics such as order entry, management, and pharmacy tracking.
- Bring videos of the clinical setting to classrooms for large group orientations, especially when orienting students to settings such as the emergency room or operating room that may be less available for student orientations.

TECHNOLOGIES IN THE HOME SETTING, TELEHEALTH, AND MORE

Learning about telehealth provides students opportunities to participate in improving patient care in the home. At a time focused on patient self-care management (IOM, Committee on the Health Professions Education, 2003), telehealth is particularly relevant. As the patient role changes to more self-directed care in the home, telehealth provides opportunities for enhanced patient care. Students need to be prepared to participate in this changing approach to health care, gaining skills in monitoring and supporting patients at a distance.

Telehealth serves as a technology tool to improve connections with patients at a distance. Telehealth does not seem foreign if one considers that telehealth is at least as old as the telephone. Phone advice services provided by urgent care health professionals or phone nurse follow-up from a physician's office are approaches everyone is familiar with. Telehealth involves understanding pathways and protocols. As people seek care in their home settings versus more structured care facilities, students learn that new technologies make this care more possible.

Whether students are assigned to work with the telehealth teams or use the equipment as part of educational activities, learning opportunities for students exist, including assisting them in learning relevant concepts. There are varied concepts and descriptors of telehealth, and, as with all technologies, the boundaries are blurring. McGonigle and Mastrian (2008) describe telehealth as including collection of clinical data for disease management, providing disease prevention programs such as asthma management, real-time video for emergent care needs, and follow-up health care services. Telehealth is often considered to include a video component and peripheral devices (such as for electronic vitals) for transmission to a central provider. The transmission of digital images such as X-rays and MRIs is another component as well. Electronic medicine, with e-mail and electronic access to practice resources, is sometimes considered in relationship to telehealth. Opportunities for earlier, more rapid assessment exist with telehealth. Telehealth involves patient follow-up and monitoring patient care beyond the hospital. From simple to complex, care is now being provided in the home and distant settings from major care providers.

Students can gain skills for assisting patients to return to their home setting. Medical management devices, sensors, and activity monitoring are tools of telehealth, providing student opportunities to learn about biometric medical devices, such as pulse oximetry, and peak flow meters as they help families learn about using these tools. Helping patients with technologies in the home can be as basic as helping manage a new hearing aid or as complex as considering a smart house or home electronic monitoring systems. These sensor technologies extend home support for patient functional deficits ranging from monitoring of wandering behaviors to electronic medication reminders.

Particularly with an aging population, there are benefits in learning about tools to help older adults remain in their homes. The IOM (2008) report on retooling for an aging America suggests that students can use technology and distance caregiving tools, learning about caregiving and gaining assessment skills in the following areas:

- Patient care needs
- Safety and functional issues in the home environment
- Informal support systems
- Community environment resources
- Cultural understanding of the caregiving context and cultural differences and preferences

Faculty can prepare students to use technologies in monitoring care and providing care at a distance. Faculty can ask students to read, review Web resources, and think creatively about how technologies can enhance safety and life quality for those individuals choosing to remain at home. Telehealth provides clinical opportunities for student learning from home settings to rural clinics and caregivers. Sample telehealth examples for education include the following:

- Monitoring a patient with a chronic illness in the home
- Teaching and monitoring health promotion plans via Web-based resources
- Providing off-site critical care monitoring by practitioners
- Treating schoolchildren with illness in partnership with a school nurse
- Providing patient education via varied online resources

Organizational resources and texts provide guidelines for additional work in this area. Further details on these topics are provided in resources such as McGonigle and Mastrian (2008) and Thede and Sewell (2009). Selected organizations providing further information on telehealth include the following:

- The American Telemedicine Association: http://www.american telemed.org/i4a/pages/index.cfm?pageid=1
- Telemedicine Information Exchange: http://tie.telemed.org/links/ specialties.asp
- American Academy of Ambulatory Care Nursing (AAACN): http://www.aaacn.org/
- Office for the Advancement of Telehealth : http://telehealth.hrsa.gov/

While telehealth is often considered in relation to individual patients, students can also learn how telehealth helps focus population health and provides communication links across states and regions. In community or population health courses, students learn about tools for knowledge access (such as community health risk assessments, disaster planning, communication, and dissemination) using an evidence base to improve response readiness.

USING TECHNOLOGY IN GUIDING PATIENT EDUCATION

Students need to be well-versed in technology that supports patient education. In a rapidly changing health care world, diverse patients cope with complex problems in less structured settings such as their homes. Technology allows more opportunities for gaining information to promote self-management. As patients assume more responsibility for their own care and well-being, one of the most important things nurses do to provide safety and quality care is patient education.

At this time of urgent need for patient education, technology offers many opportunities for supporting patients and families. It also offers many challenges as patients go to the Web and find a variety of resources, some evidence-based and many not. Students take on new roles in learning to guide their patients in appropriate uses of Web resources for health care. Learning to critique Web resources as students (as discussed in Chapter 5) now extends to helping patients learn to recognize quality Web resources when they search the Web on their own.

In addition to freely accessible health-related Web resources, a variety of clinical agencies now provide their own Web site directed toward patient support. Thede and Sewell (2009) noted these Web sites often include a variety of resources such as message boards, chat room, e-mail lists, or some combination. Sometimes online support groups are also considered within these venues, bringing their own unique issues, such as whether or not sites are moderated and who has access. Guiding students as they share evidence-based Web sites and help their patients learn basic Web site critique are beginning steps in improving patient care.

SUMMARY

Clinical experiences serve as opportunities to integrate theory into practice. Clinical faculty have the opportunity to model best practices and build student confidence and self-esteem as members of the profession. From clinical learning lab innovations with multiple types of simulations to clinical learning with varied technologies, the faculty role includes guiding students in the safe and effective use of many technologies. A focus includes monitoring of both potential and actual safety hazards in the technology-rich clinical environment.

Technology provides student learning opportunities to promote safety in the clinical settings as well as in the home. The patient care setting is where opportunities for theoretical and clinical learning come together. Best practices in clinical education with technology can help make this happen. Pedagogies of adult education and the Integrated Learning Triangle for Teaching With Technologies provide direction in both using technology and helping students learn. Teaching and learning with clinical technologies provide students opportunities for enhancing patient care.

ENDING REFLECTION

1. What is the most important content that you learned in this chapter?
2. What are your plans for using the information in this chapter in your future teaching endeavors?
3. What are your further learning goals?

GUIDELINES FOR PEDAGOGY, TECHNOLOGY, AND CLINICAL EDUCATION

Quick Tips for Clinical Teaching With Technology

1. For students new to PDA use, develop quick pocket assignments that help students gain comfort in looking up medications, unique

diagnoses, and other relevant clinical topics during any downtime in a clinical setting.
2. Use electronic concept mapping tools for students to map issues that relate to technology and patient safety.
3. Maximize student learning by reflective sharing of clinical experiences at postconference and through follow-up electronic journaling.

Questions for Further Reflection

1. What strategies can help faculty promote safe students and clinical practitioners? How much time do students need to spend in the clinical lab?
2. How do we best teach our students to gain "fingertip knowledge" with PDAs? What are the benefits and the challenges with using the Web in clinical education?
3. Should electronic devices such as PDAs be required in educational programs? What are the benefits and challenges of PDAs in promoting student independence and patient safety?

Learning Activity

What if new clinical educators headed to their first day of clinical experience with no orientation to their role, no mentor, no grading rubric, no course objectives, and no student contact information? What if they did not know how to access electronic medical records or the electronic medication system and were not sure if the group had a conference room assigned to them? What problems would exist in this scenario? If you were preparing to work with students on a new clinical unit or helping orient new faculty, how would you use technologies to help address the following questions?

1. What should I include in the students' orientation to the clinical agency?
2. How do I orient myself to the clinical agency?
3. How do I initiate and maintain good relationships with staff at the clinical agency?
4. How do I (and students) access clinical technologies such as electronic health records and medications (including needed student codes)?

Online Resources for Further Learning

■ "Medical Teamwork and Patient Safety, the Evidence-Based Relation." The Agency for Health Care Research and Quality provides this literature to promote improved patient safety: http://www.ahrq.gov/qual/medteam/

■ "Health Literacy, a Prescription to End Confusion." This IOM resource provides guidance in clear clinical communications in patient care: http://www.iom.edu/en/Reports/2004/Health-Literacy-A-Prescription-to-End-Confusion.aspx

REFERENCES

American Association of Colleges of Nursing. (2008). *The essentials of baccalaureate education for professional nursing practice.* Retrieved August 31, 2009, from http://www.aacn.nche.edu/Education/bacessn.htm

American Association of Higher Education Assessment Forum. (1993). *Nine principles of good practice for assessing student learning.* Retrieved September 12, 2009, from http://www.aahe.org/assessment/principl.htm

Benner, P., Hooper-Kyriakidis, P., & Stannard, D. (1999). *Clinical wisdom and interventions in critical care: A thinking-in-action approach.* Philadelphia: W.B. Saunders.

Galloway, S.J. (2009). Simulation techniques to bridge the gap between novice and competent healthcare professionals. *Online Journal in Nursing, 14*(2). Retrieved September 12, 2009, from http://www.nursingworld.org/MainMenuCategories/ANAMarketplace/ANAPeriodicals/OJIN.aspx

Hermann, J. (2008). *Creative teaching strategies for the nurse educator.* Philadelphia: FA Davis.

Hudson-Carlton, K., & Worrell-Carlisle, P. (2005). The learning resource center. In D. Billings & J. Halstead (Eds.), *Teaching in nursing: A guide for faculty.* St. Louis, MO: Elsevier-Saunders.

Institute of Medicine. (2008). *Retooling for an aging America: Building the health care workforce.* Retrieved October 16, 2009, from http://www.iom.edu/CMS/3809/40113/53452.aspx

Institute of Medicine Committee on the Health Professions Education. (2003). *Health professions education: A bridge to quality.* Washington, DC: The National Academies Press.

Jeffries, P. (2007). *Simulation in nursing education: From conceptualization to evaluation.* New York: NLN Publications.

McGonigle, D., & Mastrian, K. (2008). *Nursing informatics and the foundation of knowledge.* Boston, MA: Jones & Bartlett Publishers.

Thede, L., & Sewell, J. (2009). *Informatics and nursing: Competencies and applications.* Philadelphia: Lippincott.

Walvoord, B., & Anderson, V. (1998). *Effective grading: A tool for learning and assessment.* San Francisco: Jossey-Bass.

Warren, J., Meyer, M., Thompson, T., & Roche, A. (in press). Transforming nursing education: Integrating informatics and simulations. In C. Weaver, C. Delaney, P. Weber, &

R. Carr (Eds.), *Nursing and informatics for the 21st century: An international look at practice, trends and the future* (2nd ed.). Chicago: Healthcare Information and Management Systems Society.

Case Example Bibliography

Altman, T., & Brady, D. (2005). PDAs bring information competence to the point-of-care. *International Journal of Nursing Education Scholarship, 2*(1).

Cronenwett, L., Sherwood, G., Barnsteiner, J., Disch, J., Johnson, J., Mitchell, P., et al. (2007). Quality and safety education for nurses. *Nursing Outlook, 55*(3), 122–131.

Farrell, M., & Rose, L. (2008). Use of mobile handheld computers in clinical nursing education. *Journal of Nursing Education, 47*(1), 13–19.

Fisher, K., & Koren, A. (2007). Palm perspectives: The use of personal digital assistants in nursing clinical education. A qualitative study. *Online Journal of Nursing Informatics, 11*(2). Retrieved from http://ojni.org/11_2/fisher.htm

Goldsworthy, S., Lawrence, N., & Goodman, W. (2006). The use of personal digital assistants at the point of care in an undergraduate nursing program. *CIN: Computers, Informatics, Nursing, 24*, 138–143.

National League for Nursing (NLN) & University of Kansas. (2008). *HITS advancing health information technologies through faculty empowerment.* Retrieved August 8, 2008, from http://www.hits-colab.org

Rauen, C., Chulay, M., Bridges, E., Vollman, K., & Arbour, R. (2008). Seven evidence-based practice habits: Putting some sacred cows out to pasture. *Critical Care Nurse, 28*(2), 98–102.

Sorenson, D., & Dieter, C. (2005). From beginning to end: Video-based instructional and evaluation applications. *Nurse Educator, 30*(1), 40–43.

Into the Future: Nurse Educators, Teaching Technologies, and Self-Directed Lifelong Learning

CHAPTER GOAL

To be reflective educators and look toward the future with a lifelong learning frame.

BEGINNING REFLECTION

1. What are your thoughts about future pedagogies and technology and student education?
2. What learning goals will you build on to stay current?

INTRODUCTION

We are being asked to teach in ways we have not been taught and with tools we have not used. We are experiencing changing roles as faulty when we add technologies to our teaching. We negotiate new roles, sometimes dealing with internal conflict as we move from more traditional teaching methods to integrate technologies that may not even have been invented when we attended our initial nursing programs. The learning curve is large and calls for our best self-directed learning skills. The call for new skills for a new age is described by Porter-O'Grady and Malloch (2007). We negotiate new roles as we consider what technologies can be used to enhance student learning.

As noted throughout the text, change is the one certainty in the future of education. We do not know what the future holds in technology, but we can hypothesize rapid, ongoing change. When the authors started teaching, for example, the Internet had never been used in education. Preparing to teach students new technologies and to teach using new technologies in the future requires accepting that technology will change and that we will need to stay flexible. Educational technology, information management, and clinical practice technology are three frames to guide our future technology work (Skiba, Connors, & Jeffries, 2008). Identifying broad concepts and models within each of these frames helps us maintain a pedagogical base that moves us forward.

Even as we gain a tool set for teaching with technologies, technology will continue to change, with many further means emerging to promote student learning. The teacher as learner gains a synthesis of key points from this text as the basis for further projects, recalling in particular that traditional pedagogies and emerging educational best practices help guide our work. This book has provided a collage of skills and thoughts for taking us into our changing classroom and clinical settings. Reflecting on the concepts in this book assists in planning the use of technology in our classrooms. This chapter reminds us to be reflective educators, to collaborate in future learning practices, and to look toward the future with a lifelong learning frame.

BEING A REFLECTIVE EDUCATOR

A reflective educator looks back and considers what has or has not been accomplished. A reflective educator is one who makes teaching and learning visible or clearly communicates the work of educators to others. Bernstein, Burnett, Goodburn, and Savory (2006) reflect on the importance of documenting what we do as teachers to help our learners achieve. As faculty we can name what we do, considering what has worked well and what needs further work in our teaching and learning projects.

Readers are reminded of self-directed learning and lifelong learning concepts. We cannot prepare students well for the future unless we incorporate into our teaching the current technologies they will need to function in their profession and in the future. Our text has provided a toolkit of approaches for teaching technologies and teaching our students about technologies.

Are We Teaching by the Evidence?

Models to Guide

The Integrated Learning Triangle (Appendix B), introduced in this text, has the advantages of showing quick reminders of key pieces that need to fit into teaching with technology considerations and lesson planning. As suggested in this model, opportunities exist for building on current best educational practices as well as contributing to these best practices.

Evidence-Based Teaching

While health care professionals want best evidence for clinical practice, faculty also need an evidence base for their pedagogy or teaching practice. Best teaching requires us to give thoughtful attention to the ways that we structure our teaching and learning methods to ensure that we are basing our practices on the best evidence. Specific teaching concepts, such as concept mapping or problem-based learning, can be reviewed to identify the evidence base. Oermann (2009) notes the need for research to further develop the body of literature for health professions educators and suggests some beginning approaches.

Contributing to the Evidence and Sharing Our Successes

While teaching by the evidence has been emphasized throughout the text, we also need to focus on our own educational scholarship and opportunities to contribute to best teaching practices and the generation of further educational research questions. The National League for Nursing (NLN, 2003) nurse educator competencies include sharing through scholarship as a major competency. We have as much responsibility to share our successful teaching strategies as we do our research studies. With the rapid pace of change, there is a particular need for sharing evaluative projects at this time.

Boyer's (1990) classic framework provides direction in documenting our educational scholarship. Known as the scholarship of teaching and learning (SOTL), Boyer's work acknowledges faculty educational scholarship as well as faculty clinical research. His framework is based on teaching, application, integration, and discovery. Specific to application scholarship, for example, faculty might develop an online learning object or activity, implement and evaluate it, and then share it for others to learn from. A process of naming and packaging the object or activity, having it peer reviewed, and then publishing it for others to learn from (Huber & Hutchings, 2005) provides the application of scholarship. Technology teaching and learning repositories and online educational journals make it easier than ever to share our products with diverse audiences.

Scholarship of Teaching and Learning as Quality Improvement

The increased use of technology has pushed us to examine how we teach. This scholarship approach also engages us as reflective educators and provides a form of continuous quality improvement as we reflect on what we have done and then strive to continuously make our teaching better. Opportunities for teaching with technology provide an excellent time to examine the quality of our teaching work. Creating one's own quality improvement is as basic as reflecting on process and outcomes in our courses. We can use tools such as satisfaction surveys that are already in place. Questions are tools to keep us thinking and moving forward in our quality

Exhibit 15.1

BENEFITS TO THE SCHOLARSHIP OF TEACHING AND LEARNING (SOTL) PROJECTS

- The scholarship of teaching and learning provides rich representation/description of our educational projects.
- Evaluation/evidence can lead to generating new project questions and questions for further educational research.
- Benefits of being reflective educational practitioners are evident and include opportunities for self-assessment and ongoing quality improvement in our teaching.
- Faculty gain opportunities to share and learn from each other's projects; the sharing can help create a learning community in our programs.
- Faculty gain the opportunity to organize/document our teaching protocols, to name what it is we do.
- The scholarship of teaching and learning demonstrates our thoughtful attention to our teaching and our efforts to continue to improve our practices within our changing nursing student populations and programs.

improvement. Generating good questions is a part of effective reflective practice, helping us guide our planning (what is working) as well as to consider opportunities for further study. Particularly with our rapidly changing technology world, questions provide guidance in the many areas that will continue to evolve.

SOTL supports a spirit of inquiry to guide us into the future. Technology projects serve as excellent exemplars for scholarly projects. Publishing our work helps others learn from our challenges and gain from our successes in projects specific to teaching with technologies. This provides a way to pass on what we have learned about teaching and educational best practices. If we are not sharing our own learning, it can be lost. See Exhibit 15.1 on further benefits to SOTL.

COLLABORATING FOR FUTURE LEARNING GOALS

Gaining Mentorship and Being a Mentor

As many faculty have had few role models for teaching with technology, a steep learning curve exists without a mentor to guide us. Trusted principles and theories serve well, but mentors, as wise and trusted counselors, also champion our work with technology. Learning about rapidly emerging technology often involves finding champions of specific technology approaches and learning from these mentors. Gaining a mentor who is willing to share teaching tips or conversation on selected teaching with technology projects can enhance our work.

Mentors can now be more than local individuals, since we are all able to access individuals electronically whether nearby or at a distance. Finding a local mentor often involves asking those whose work we admire. Having a plan for how to ask for what is needed, such as follow-up conversations and assessments, is key as well. Finding a mentor at a distance is often facilitated by national programs such as Health Information Technology Scholars Program (HITS) and the NLN mentoring programs. Both programs serve as examples of mentoring at a national level where prominent individuals provide guidance in selected project work. Guides are available with tips for setting up mentoring plans, both as a mentor and as a mentee (NLN, 2006; Zachary, 2000).

Other options for mentoring include informal mentoring opportunities and peer group mentoring. Informal mentoring, for example, can be gained from the literature, following the works of experts in our technology area of interest. Often text authors provide additional journal articles or online resources for review. Peer groups can serve a supportive and encouraging function as local faculty members become learning partners in working on a technology project together. Developing a peer group of technology champions can promote enthusiasm and creativity in developing course projects. Tools such as the New Technology Readiness Inventory (Appendix A) and the Integrated Learning Triangle (Appendix B) can provide direction.

Technology, Pedagogy, and Interdisciplinary Clinical Partners

Teaching with technology is not a solitary endeavor in health care. Working and learning collaboratively with interdisciplinary colleagues and clinical partners benefits students' learning for future practice. Institute of Medicine (IOM, 2003) reports recommend using technology and working as interdisciplinary teams to further clinical learning goals. Interdisciplinary education involves two or more academic disciplines. Learning as teams can help students gain beginning insights into various team members' perceptions of their role in practice. In the same way, faculty can partner to learn from what other disciplines are doing in technology-related pedagogies.

Partnering with other health care professions for traditional interdisciplinary classroom education is a strategy that some have found challenging. Diverse campus settings, diverse semester and clinical schedules, and increased faculty responsibilities are sample challenges. Problems can exist—for example, finding common settings and times to hold interdisciplinary classes. An option that avoids the time and space classroom challenges involves partnering to develop and deliver interdisciplinary continuing education via the Web. Online asynchronous technology is especially useful at a time when schedules can make getting students from different disciplines together difficult. Product Web reviews can also provide an interdisciplinary component.

Additionally, high-fidelity simulation technology has become increasingly popular in providing new opportunities for interdisciplinary education. Opportunities with simulators include learning improved communication modes and gaining insight into the perspectives of other disciplines. These learning opportunities also provide a broader systems approach to learning that avoids compartmentalization of basic science, behavioral science, and clinical disciplines as recommended by the IOM (2003) health pro-

Exhibit 15.2

SHARING INTERDISCIPLINARY RESOURCES

Sample learning opportunities for working as part of interdisciplinary teams include the following:

- *Classroom and online learning opportunities.* One way to promote interdisciplinary education includes extending collaborative learning efforts via technology. McGonigle and Mastrian (2009) note that informatics concepts and courses are well suited to interdisciplinary education. Working as teams and utilizing informatics are two of the recommended competencies from IOM (2003).
- *Sharing interdisciplinary resources online.* Sharing interdisciplinary resources for critique exposes nurses to new ways of approaching problems as we learn about tools of the various disciplines.
- *Safety projects and interdisciplinary learning.* Technology plays a central role in providing better communication and promoting a safer patient care environment. With the focus on safe, quality care, the entire health care team is engaged, including the patient as part of that team. Our range for safety is broad, from infant safety teaching to helping older adults manage complex medication regimens. Our guiding assignment question might be, "How can students best learn to engage with patients, staff, students, and others in participating as members of the safety health care team?"

fessions educator report. This report also notes that further development of what works in clinical education is needed, including the determination of what content matters most and what teaching strategies work best. Students' care of a variety of clients, in a variety of settings, can only be enhanced through better understanding roles of multiple disciplines. Exhibit 15.2 provides sample learning opportunities for working as part of interdisciplinary teams.

TEACHING WITH TECHNOLOGIES: INTO THE FUTURE

As both educators and learners we will need to stay motivated and continue to be self-directed learners if we are to keep up with this rapidly changing technology and the pace of clinical education. Varied learning approaches can be combined to help us keep up with ongoing and future changes. Future learning includes accessing just-in-time resources. For example, online tutorials or freely accessible online videos as well as traditional written materials are extensive. Just-in-time education is no longer simply nice to have but is often required on a regular basis. Sample suggestions for creating learning plans include the following:

- Gain Web education, both formal and informal, including both pedagogical and clinical resources.
- Create informal learning plans based on trusted clinical organizational resources.
- Seek resources from national leadership in the clinical education arena, such as Technology Informatics Guiding Educational Reform (TIGER), Quality and Safety Education for Nurses (QSEN), and the Health Information Technology Scholars (HITS) program.
- Seek out resources from professional nursing or interdisciplinary associations, such as the American Nurses Association or the American Geriatrics Society.
- Keep up via listservs and other electronic networks in an area of specialty interest.
- Attend actual or virtual meetings.
- Scan program topics from online conference brochures.
- Participate in learning object repositories such as the Teaching, Learning, and Technology Group (http://www.tltgroup.org/) and others.
- Continue formal coursework, such as courses on teaching with technologies (Bonnel, Wambach, & Connors, 2005).
- Mentor others by working with technology-invested younger faculty to blend seasoned educators' years of pedagogical experience with their enthusiasm for technology (or vice versa).
- Scan for current trends that influence and guide teaching with various technologies. A reflective educator scans the horizon and thinks about what is needed to stay current.
- Participate in national task forces. Opportunities that might previously have been cost-prohibitive—to participate in state, national, and international organizations and their task groups—can now be accomplished from the comfort of work or home offices.

CHANGING OUR EDUCATION TO FIT THE CHANGING WORLD

Looking back to the IOM reports serves as a reminder of the important role educators have to play. These reports are key components in the current restructuring of health care; an important element of this restructuring

Exhibit 15.3

INSTITUTE OF MEDICINE HEALTH PROFESSIONS EDUCATION REVISITED

IOM (2003) provides faculty with direction in moving nursing education forward. *Technology* serves in uniting the IOM concepts, including the following examples:

- **Interdisciplinary practice.** Clinical team members are brought together in new ways to share data management via electronic health records and diverse technologies such as simulation labs and Web-based programs.
- **Evidence-based practice.** Technology serves as a central tool in search, access, critique, and synthesis of best evidence for practice. It helps move evidence to protocol formats that can be electronically shared, used, and evaluated.
- **Information management in quality improvement.** Informatics tools help in designing individual and population databases that serve the needs of patients, providers, and other health care system team members.
- **Client-centered care.** Care advances such as electronic information systems and the Web help enhance the patient as the center of the team, giving him or her access to data and resources for informed clinical decisions.

is to eliminate gaps between education and practice. Health care provider education includes not only focusing on the reports' content but also incorporating core competencies, including safety and quality care. This book has been about using technology to help us do this. See Exhibit 15.3 for a summary related to the IOM (2003) and health professions report.

Change is the one certainty in the future of education. What is cutting-edge today will quickly pass, replaced by newer technology. Technology has provided new ways to envision our teaching/learning approaches to help students gain needed competencies. As our younger, technology-savvy students move into clinical practice, they will be prepared to learn and build with technology resources. Examples of the ways in which students will use new technology include the following:

- Gaining experiences with PDA-type devices for keeping up with the evidence needed in their patients' care.
- Building opportunities for learning with the Web and not just within the confines of an online course to gain evidence-based resources for the future.
- Gaining confidence for their patient care responsibilities and future staff development roles in using high-tech simulators.
- Learning skills in data management to promote the health of the populations they care for.

Exhibit 15.4

GUIDELINES FOR SHARING THE SCHOLARSHIP OF TECHNOLOGY PROJECTS

To share an assignment or teaching project, use a project summary format that might be used in developing a professional portfolio or in beginning steps for manuscript development. The descriptive sharing will include not only the assignment/project structure but also the challenges, strategies, process, and outcomes. For example, consider the following questions:

- What is the assignment/project about?
- Why is it important?
- How is it designed (the structure, the process)?
- How do faculty and students participate or process roles?
- How are students evaluated? What are the outcomes?
- On completion, what was especially good or challenging about the project? What would you do differently next time?

Preparing to teach with technologies in the future requires accepting that technology will change and that we will need to stay flexible. Selected take-home points from this chapter include the following:

- Use lifelong learning as more than a buzzword.
- Build bridges with interdisciplinary practice partners.
- Gain a mentor and community network of fellow learners.
- Identify strategies to scan the future and keep up.
- Evaluate what does and does not work in teaching with technologies for selected populations.
- Contribute to the scholarship of teaching, learning, and sharing best practices.

Sharing a teaching with technology project as scholarship, as previously noted, provides a way to continue learning and promotes quality in our teaching. Exhibit 15.4 provides ideas for a beginning write-up of a teaching project.

SUMMARY

Basic educational principles do not change as we move into teaching with technologies. Building on an evidence base and guiding our work with best practices and relevant theory direct our teaching activities. Technology challenges us but also provides the potential to ease selected challenges in education of the future. Teaching with technology into the future is not a race that one should try to win. It relates more to pacing ourselves and building on solid pedagogies in helping students via educational technologies, clinical technologies, and informatics. In all cases, our goals continue to include developing professional, competent students prepared to enhance patient care.

ENDING REFLECTION

1. What is the most important content that you learned in this chapter?
2. What are your plans for using the information in this chapter in your future teaching endeavors?
3. What are your further learning goals?

GUIDELINES FOR INTO THE FUTURE: NURSE EDUCATORS, TEACHING TECHNOLOGIES, AND SELF-DIRECTED LIFELONG LEARNING

Quick Tips for Using Technology Into the Future

1. Consider roles and responsibilities in mentoring and being mentored.
2. Implement a portfolio project that showcases a teaching with technology assignment or class as a way to demonstrate educational scholarship.
3. Gain skills in peer review and project dissemination in sharing scholarship of teaching with technologies.

Questions for Reflection

1. What strategies do we as educators need to consider to be a proactive rather than reactive part of the future?
2. What strategies can help us make the SOTL more a part of our professional teaching careers or clinical educator roles?

Learning Activity

As a reflective educator, consider the following reflective prompts to assist in further planning with technologies.

1. What are your best successes in teaching with technologies? What is working best for you in teaching or learning with technology?
2. What are your biggest concerns in teaching with technologies? What questions/topics do you have to plan for?
3. What are examples of technology projects that you have successfully shared? What made that happen? What factors could further encourage and support professional sharing?

Online Resources for Further Learning

- Tomorrow's Professor listserv. This ongoing listserv provides continued ideas for improving pedagogical skills: http://ctl.stanford.edu/Tomprof/postings.html
- "Emerging Perspectives on Learning, Teaching, and Technology." This online text, edited by Michael Orey, provides an example of an ongoing text development process as well as a text used for multiple purposes and should provide reading into the future: http://projects.coe.uga.edu/epltt/index.php?title=Main_Page

REFERENCES

Bernstein, D., Burnett, A., Goodburn, A., & Savory, P. (2006). *Making teaching and learning visible: Course portfolios and the peer review of teaching.* San Francisco: Jossey-Bass.

Bonnel, W., Wambach, K., & Connors, H. (2005). A nurse educator teaching with technologies course: More than teaching on the Web. *Journal of Professional Nursing, 21*(1), 59–65.

Boyer, E. L. (1990). *Scholarship reconsidered: Priorities of the professoriate.* Princeton, NJ: Carnegie Foundation for the Advancement of Teaching.

Huber, M., & Hutchings, P. (2005). *The advancement of learning: Building the teaching commons.* San Francisco: Jossey-Bass.

Institute of Medicine. (2003). *Health professions education: A bridge to quality.* Washington, DC: National Academies Press.

McGonigle, D., & Mastrian, K. (2009). *Nursing informatics and the foundation of knowledge.* Boston: Jones & Bartlett Publishers.

National League for Nursing. (2003). *Core competencies of nurse educators.* Retrieved October 16, 2009, from http://www.nln.org/profdev/corecompletter.htm

National League for Nursing. (2006). *Mentoring position statement.* Retrieved October 16, 2009, from http://www.nln.org/aboutnln/PositionStatements/mentoring_3_21_06.pdf

Oermann, M. (2009). *Evidence-based nursing education, leader to leader—National Council of State Boards of Nursing.* Retrieved October 16, 2009, from https://www.ncsbn.org/Leader-to-Leader_Spring09.pdf

Porter-O'Grady, T., & Malloch, K. (2007). *Quantum leadership: A resource for health care innovation* (2nd ed.). Boston: Jones & Bartlett.

Skiba, D.J., Connors, H.R., & Jeffries, P. (2008). Information technologies and the transformation of nursing education. *Nursing Outlook, 56*(5), 225–230.

Zachary, L.J. (2000). *The mentor's guide: Facilitating effective learning relationships.* San Francisco: Jossey-Bass.

APPENDIX A

New Technology Readiness Inventory

The following inventory can help answer the why, how, and when of learning a new technology. Organized around the concepts of readiness, opportunity, and support, the inventory provides direction in identifying an individualized plan. Please reflect on the following items specific to a new technology you would like to teach with.

1. For the *specific* technology, what is your:
   a. Readiness/motivation—What is your readiness to learn/gain comfort with the technology? Would you rate this as low, moderate, or high?
   b. Opportunity—What is available to you in terms of technology resources and environment? Are there opportunities to access the technology you hope to use?
   c. Support—Who is available (locally or at a distance) to mentor or coach you in teaching with a specific technology?
2. Based on your assessment, what learning goals will you set?
   Goal statement (includes your intention and time frame):

3. Based on your goals, what specific plan will you design to enhance your technology learning/comfort needs?

    Plan (includes two to three specific action steps):

4. What potential challenges exist or might limit your efforts? What strategies would be most likely to promote success?

Integrated Learning Triangle for Teaching With Technologies

The following guides flow from the Integrated Learning Triangle for Teaching With Technologies and can help answer the why, how, and when of using technology for a specific course, lesson, or assignment. Questions are organized around the mnemonic BEBOLDER to guide reflection. Consider the following items as you think about your plans for using technology.

- **Best practices.** What evidence is available to guide implementing a particular technology? What are recommended approaches?
- **Educational principles and theories.** What broad principles or theories such as adult education theory best fit student learning needs and teaching opportunities?
- **Beginning assessments.** What are student learning needs specific to the student level and content to be taught?
- **Objectives.** What is to be achieved in a specific course, lesson, or assignment? How can technology help?
- **Logistics/context.** What is the setting for teaching/learning? What physical resources are available? What are student numbers and available resource people to assist?
- **Decision/fit.** What is the best technology fit for given learning needs and resources?

<u>Integrated Learning Triangle for Teaching with Technologies</u>

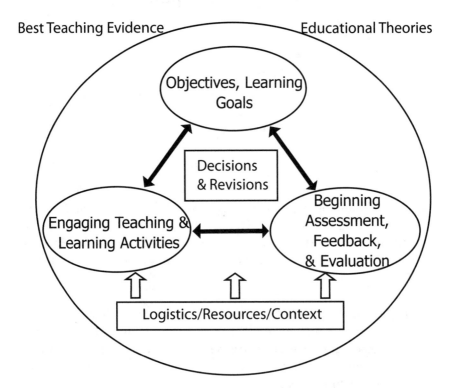

- **Evaluation and feedback.** What is the evaluation plan? What feedback mechanisms are integrated into the course? How will you know if technology is helping students learn?
- **Review and revision.** How will you build quality improvement into your plan? What worked and what did not? What needs to be improved?

FURTHER QUESTIONS TO GUIDE REFLECTIONS

How does a particular technology best meet learning needs? For a particular course or assignment, will the technology:

- Help capture the concepts you are teaching?
- Assist students in meeting the objectives of the course?
- Help focus students' learning? Motivate students to become involved in learning?
- Help students make transitions to practice or focus on important concepts?

Also, for a given point in time:

- Is a particular technology worth the time and effort? (Would a less expensive technology work as well? What are the trade-offs?)
- What is the evidence for using the technology? (If there is limited evidence, is it consistent with good theory and educational principles?)
- Is the workload reasonable and well placed for both faculty and students?

Index